I0152302

HE'S NOT MAD, HE'S MY BROTHER

MARC GRAHAM KING

WINNER OF THE NATIONAL SPIRITUAL WRITING COMPETITION

Marc Graham King © 2024

All rights reserved in accordance with the Copyright, Designs and Patents Act 1988.

No parts of this publication may be reproduced, stored in a retrieval system, or transmitted in any form or by any means whatsoever without the prior permission of the publisher.

A record of this publication is available from the British Library.

ISBN 978-1-910027-63-9

Typesetting and cover design by Titanium Design Ltd

https://www.titaniumdesign.co.uk

Cover image licensed by https://www.mgkdesign.co.uk

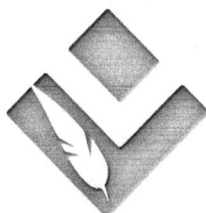

**LOCAL
LEGEND**

Published by Local Legend
https://local-legend.co.uk

DEDICATION

To my brother, Jason. Thank you for your help in writing this book. I dearly hope that in turn it helps you to achieve your dream of preventing others from living a life of addiction and encouraging them to seek help. They will know that they have your heartfelt understanding.

ACKNOWLEDGEMENTS

My love of words was inspired by a dedicated teacher, Mike Smith, who introduced me to English Literature when I was a troubled teenager attending a rough London comprehensive school. Mike's patient enthusiasm and encouragement opened the door to an enthralling new world and I want his family to know how much I shall always cherish his memory.

I am also deeply grateful to Mabel, my loyal and ancient Frenchie, for always recognising when I'm too busy and stressed and insisting on taking a walk. She has taught me to stop and take a breath, and has shown me the magic of everyday life.

https://local-legend.co.uk

ABOUT THE AUTHOR

Marc Graham King lives in south-west London, UK, and runs his own creative design company. His love of literature was inspired by a school teacher, later leading to a writing course and a decade-long passion for pursuing his dream of becoming an author.

His inspirations are the science fiction and fantasy of David Mitchell and John Wyndham and contemporary writing masters such as Grahame Greene, Brian Moore, Chris Cleave and Andrew Miller.

Throughout his life, Marc has had a close and loving relationship with his younger brother, yet was powerless to prevent Jason's descent into drug addiction. It is a familiar story for so many families these days. However, Marc has never hesitated to support and care for his brother.

This memoir, written with Jason's collaboration, is searingly honest and deeply compassionate. It shows us all how fragile our mental health can be and how very easy it is to lose our way. And it shines a clear spotlight on the deficiencies of our national health services.

Marc's website is https://www.marcgrahamking.com

Previous Publications

Gangster Farm (Amazon Kindle Edition, 2018)

CONTENTS

INTRODUCTION

"There are three sides to every story.
Yours. Mine. What really happened."
(Jeyn Roberts, *Rage Within*)

You only have to look at my brother to see he's an addled druggie. Six feet one and nine and a half stone, scrawny and emaciated, he personifies turmoil. Now in his fifties, his shoulder-length hair is usually tangled, oily or matted. If I point this out, he ignores me. Yet should I point out the greyness, he protests vehemently, "I'm not going fucking grey." There are things I can see that my brother clearly can't, and perhaps vice versa.

When Jason protests fervently like this, I can still recognise within his pale blue eyes remnants of normality despite his tattered years of self-neglect, first experimenting with drugs at the age of fourteen.

And somewhere in the quietness of my mind, I have to confess that there is something compulsive about his claims that he's been plagued by supernatural visitations since childhood. He's adamant there's legitimate evidence to back him up too.

"I'm telling you, Marc," he'll say pleadingly as if repeating this somehow makes it all true. "These things follow me about. I'm telling the truth."

To a stranger, his claim probably sound ludicrous. It's difficult to fathom and to treat seriously and I can only listen with the care of a man who loves his unsound brother. There's one nagging question for me, though: was the moment he entered our strange new home,

Fir Tree Cottage, at age four the catalyst for all his trauma?

Our mother had another theory when I discussed Jason with her.

"He was a footling." She drained the last of the wine from her glass and moved towards the fridge for a top-up with a furrowed expression. "Breech babies arriving feet first can receive brain damage during birth," she continued. "He couldn't walk until he was eighteen months." Perched on the corner of the kitchen table she pondered this fact ruefully, gazing through the window as her cigarette smoke curled through the air. "On the other hand, he could say multi-syllable words like elephant and hippopotamus long before you could utter basic ones."

Yet I always knew Jason wasn't 'backward'. He was intelligent at school, a thoughtful boy who pondered rather than squandered his words. My brother was profoundly creative, always excelling at art. I think our mother was clutching at straws.

The unavoidable truth is that no single fact has ever been able to explain my younger brother.

My attempts to tell Jason's story may sound at times like fantasy or warped memory. But the events I'm writing about actually did happen. I've long been Jason's carer and loving brother and I have researched others' personal accounts. These include those chronicled in the eminent Catholic priest Dom Robert Petitpierre's memoir, *Exorcising Devils,* the relevance of which will become clear.

My hope is that if you ever come across a person like my brother, someone with mental health and addiction issues, you will try to consider their back story. The past unavoidably moulds our future, sometimes in small ways, sometimes shaping our entire existence. And in Jason's history, there is that extra paranormal factor that we have never been able to explain.

1

THE BIRTHDAY

"Thanks for letting me stay, Marc. You're a good brother."

Slouched in an armchair, Jason spoke without turning his face from the TV documentary on alien visitations. After a month-long bender with his girlfriend, he had come to stay with me for a few days. His stopovers were never entirely pleasurable but they always had their brotherly moments.

"Diane loved watching alien conspiracies," he mumbled, the corner of his eyes glinting with emotion.

"So are you two finished, Jason?"

"I don't know. I just needed to get out. We're bad for each other, you know. Two addicts should never be together, it's a fucking disaster." He turned towards me with a hopeless, craggy smile.

When he was lucid and measured like this, it rejuvenated the strong friendship we'd shared as children. With his bender behind him, my real brother returned. How long this would last was always impossible to estimate.

"I'll do the washing up, Marc. Let me help with things around the house. I owe you."

Jason was always kind and considerate. And right now he was easier to converse with than the frightened wreck who'd arrived at my house bewildered and upset. He was happier and again characteristically chirpy as he played with the kids, the comfortable disorder of a normal home life reviving his normality.

"You don't owe me anything," I reassured him. "I want to help."

He was completely broke and I needed to help him find somewhere to live until we could hopefully arrange permanent council accommodation. I had no space for him long term and felt anxious leaving him alone during the day in the same way you wouldn't leave a six year-old child alone with matches.

It was an ongoing struggle to secure state accommodation for him and all I could really do was vet anywhere he found to the best of my ability in my new role as his temporary housing officer. I was mindful of finding a place where the other tenants weren't simply interested in selling his CDs or using his mattress to hide their works.

"We'll find somewhere, Jason. But wherever we find needs to be safer than the last place."

"That shouldn't be too hard," he snorted indignantly, still watching avidly as some fake flying saucer shot across the screen.

Jason was in a happier mood. I'd lifted his spirits by arranging a pub get-together to celebrate his birthday with my friends. I'd also slipped him forty quid along with his birthday presents of new clothes and a pair of smart boots he'd asked for. I admit this filled me with unease; putting money in his pocket was dangerous as I knew how he liked to spend his cash.

Waiting at the bar alone, I felt a rush of relief as the pub door swung open with a rush of cold winter air. My friends entered full of high spirits. Approaching the bar, Tony looked around at the milling crowd.

"Busy for a Wednesday, isn't it?" he asked.

This was normally a quiet pub at seven-thirty mid-week and the five of us vied for attention from the barmaids, each of us insisting on getting the first round. We'd been friends since school and the familiar banter was always easy. I nodded towards the far corner of the pub where Jason slouched in an armchair by the fireplace, his face lit by the flickering flames. The laughter stopped. With his head slumped and four empty pint glasses lined up neatly on the table, the occasional lolling of his head was the only clue to life.

"Thanks for coming," I told my friends with poorly concealed melancholy. I was indeed grateful that they often turned up for my brother's birthdays, since who else would bother? The only friends Jason had were fellow addicts. Even then, those he declared his friends were only ever names and unseen faces he'd known slightly for a few weeks.

"Dave, he's a great bloke… John, he's my best mate…"

And predictably these names would disappear as quickly as his DVDs, his loose change and his CD player. They were counterfeit friends who placated him with companionship then pissed on his sofa, stole his minimal possessions and betrayed all his hopes of real friendship.

"How long have you been here?" Tony asked me, still staring across at Jason.

"About forty-five minutes," I said, and we began to laugh.

With customary pragmatism, Richard observed, "He'd better slow down or I'll never catch up."

"Come on, say hello to the birthday boy."

We threaded our way through the growing number of punters towards my brother's table. Darren nudged Jason's arm and presented him with a smile and a fresh pint of cider.

"Happy birthday, mate," he said with a caring smile.

"Thaaan you," Jason slurred, smiling at the friendly face with brief if confused recognition. Pushing himself upright he grinned, taking a big gulp of his pint before slumping back into his chair and closing his eyes contentedly.

"Yeah, Jason. Happy birthday, you old git. How old are you today anyway?" Darryl gave his hand a friendly squeeze, although clearly shocked by my brother's deteriorated appearance.

"Aaash old aaash my tongue an' a bit older'n my teeth," Jason jibed with a wry smile, eyes still shut.

The pub door opened and closed continuously and soon the place was uncomfortably full as regulars began congregating into small groups, commandeering all available tables and perches. Papers and pens were being distributed to tables and the noisy movement suddenly froze as an amplified voice sliced through the din.

"Welcome to the Wednesday quiz night!"

I hadn't expected this, not being a regular, and I had a sudden sense of foreboding. "Tonight's first question is—"

In an instant, Jason was suddenly reanimated. Sitting bolt upright in his armchair he faced the surrounding crowd with eyes wide, red and bleary as he slammed his half-empty glass on the table.

"WHERE ARE ALL THE WHORES?" he shouted, before gulping the rest of his cider and disappearing back down into the armchair with a satisfied smile.

"I think we'd better leave," I said, looking with horror at the faces of confused punters exchanging those awkward glances, unsure how to respond. In silent agreement, the five of us drained our glasses, dragged Jason up and stumbled out into the cold, wintery night. Partially supported by my friends, Jason tried coordinating his legs along the road with a look of desperate concentration.

Irritated, I began to chastise my brother. His faltering progress was an embarrassment and how he'd become paralytic in such a short time was beyond belief.

"Come on, Jason. For heaven's sake, it'll be closing time soon."

"I was just asking about the women, Marc. It's my birthday after all, isn't it?" he shrugged, bewildered. Observing our looks of disbelief, his displeasure with himself was tangible. My friends might have still held out hope for an enjoyable night but my own hopes had been obliterated.

We made our way slowly along the soaking pavement towards a larger, more boisterous, well-known drinkers' pub where I felt confident Jason would feel more at home and where we wouldn't have to worry about any further embarrassing antics. My reasoning was that 'They're all pissheads in there anyway.'

I glanced back to check on my flagging brother, a staggering tragedy I found difficult to watch, and a surge of guilt for my earlier outburst overwhelmed me. I hated myself, especially because I'd done it in the company of others on his birthday and I'd hurt him. The more self-conscious Jason grew, the more emotional he became, his eyes tearful. I could read his inner turmoil and angst so well. Car headlights illuminated his sunken face along with his absolute displeasure with himself and his entire troubled passage through life.

"What's the latest on him getting rehab or whatever?" Darren asked with concern, glancing intermittently at Jason's slow progress.

I tried explaining the complex processes involved in securing funded rehabilitation, procedures laced with a raft of protocols that had to be strictly adhered to before consideration will even be given for costly residential treatment. I couldn't pay for it myself, with a family to support, and I was having to learn to cope with all these frustrations. Meanwhile, Jason was attending a drugs and alcohol centre that just might possibly help him secure a rehab place.

Behind us, Jason stopped to roll a cigarette, leaning against the bus stop. Passing headlights illuminated his spindly legs, casting a silhouette of tragedy across the pavement.

Jason was registered with social services as a multi-addict with underlying psychiatric problems, issues that still needed to be fully explored and investigated by professionals. Therein lay the proverbial spanner in the works. Most rehabilitation facilities won't take a candidate with suspected psychiatric problems as they could jeopardise the recovery of other residents. Rehab was always a precarious game of risk, so why make it more so if it can be avoided. This, I explained soberly to my friends, was "…another fucking obstacle to overcome…" if my brother was ever going to get professional help.

"To be honest, I don't think they really know how to handle him or what to do. He says he has strange visitations… hears voices and sees things. But he's not nuts," I reassured them, wanting to lift the hopelessness on their faces. "He's got issues, they believe, from when we were kids."

My friends were familiar with our family history. They'd known my brother for many years and had been witness to his progressive decline. They remembered the whimsical schoolboy, the gangly kid who was thoughtful, intelligent and sensitive. My brother didn't have lots of friends at school but they knew he had no enemies either.

"Have they any ideas about what's wrong with his head?" Paul asked pragmatically as we waited for Jason to stagger the last few yards to the pub unaided and oblivious to our deliberations.

Painfully, I explained that the professionals couldn't really get a clear picture about any underlying mental problems because he masked himself with drink and drugs, some illegal, others prescription pacifiers. In order to placate him, doctors had inadvertently complicated the matter by prescribing his drug cocktail, hoping it would alleviate his appetite for Class A.

"The problem is, no-one has much time for people with mental illness, it's completely under-resourced and requires too much intervention, time and money. You get your ten minutes with the doctor, then collect your prescription. That's how it works these days."

"That's ridiculous," Darryl said, struggling to understand this lack of care and turning to my other friends who nodded in agreement.

"He's trying to come off heroin now," I continued. "He says he doesn't use intravenously anymore, he's been given Methadone instead." According to Jason, he was now just 'an occasional dabbler', whatever that meant. He'd tried convincing me this was the absolute truth but the bruised track marks on his arms and hands told a different story.

"Anyway," I eyed the pub's swing doors, determined to rescue the night, "apart from all that, he's an upstanding, well-integrated member of society." We shared a bout of ironic laughter. "But if he can't walk in by himself, there's no way we can let him continue to drink," I said, more as a plea for support than an instruction. I felt vulnerable, foolish, uncomfortable disclosing so much personal information, even to close friends.

The noise inside was harsh. Two men standing by a fruit machine were arguing over the result of a football match. A girl behind the bar dropped a glass and was met with raucous cheers. Walking to the bar with Darren, I brushed past a man standing in front of his group of friends, telling one of them repeatedly that he was a wanker while he spilled beer onto the dark, heavily stained carpet.

Jason ambled among chairs and tables looking around at faces to see if he recognised anybody or if anybody recognised him.

"There's a table at the back," Tony said. We walked over to a booth where a large table was pushed up against a boarded window decorated with several lumps of dried chewing gum. I guided Jason into the corner next to the window and sat close by, trying to include him in every facet of our discussions. It was fruitless, he remained monosyllabic, the occasional grunt or incoherent statement his only contribution as he studied his empty glass.

"My shout, I'll get some more drinks," said Paul, heading to the bar with Richard and Darryl and leaving us to watch Jason prepare another roll-up.

"He once told me," Darren said quietly, "about an old man he saw in the cottage you two used to live in." He explained it had been a good few years ago and he'd only really listened to Jason's tale out of politeness. "It was one of the few genuine conversations I've ever had with him. I didn't realise he believes all that stuff is real." He'd also told Darren about seeing other strange manifestations as a child, like light orbs outside his bedroom window at Fir Tree Cottage.

"He still has strange experiences," I said. "And he believes his girlfriend Diane has as well. It's odd really. Although he often can't remember yesterday particularly well, there are things from our past he appears to remember perfectly."

"Jason talked about objects moving in his bedroom and that he'd been physically moved himself, pulled from his bed to the floor several times," said Darren. "I just let him talk. I remember thinking it was strange, him telling me that story, being as straight as he was at the time."

I admired Darren's open-minded approach, never judging Jason or mocking him about the legitimacy of his tales. Although I'll admit his stories were occasionally pretty thought-provoking, I'd mostly dismissed them as the regurgitated fantasies of a confused mind. 'Fact or acid flashback?' was the question I always debated with myself whenever Jason confided about one of his 'occurrences'.

My own philosophy about my brother's mental health was mostly based on nurture. Some time after our father moved out, my mother had entertained an eclectic series of boyfriends, from the bohemian to the potentially brutal. I wondered whether Jason had been bullied in the same way I was, by one unsavoury character. A carpet salesman from East London, a wide boy with a pot of gold (that the taxman didn't know about) and a house in the country, this man just liked to fight and fuck. One time, the bastard had grabbed me by the throat, telling me to fuck off as he was busy upstairs with my mother. I was nine.

When it was my round, Darren and Paul came to the bar with me, leaving Jason half asleep on the table.

"He's seriously unwell now." I cupped my hands to Darren's ear to be heard above the din, all good humour now drained from my voice. "Mum told me the doctors don't think he can carry on much longer. He's got pericarditis, something to do with inflammation of the sac surrounding the heart. The substance abuse has taken its toll." I swallowed the dregs from my glass.

"That explains why you're desperate to get him help." Darren glanced back at my brother, looking as worried as I felt.

I tilted my mouth towards his ear again and repeated what the doctor, a friend of the family, had told my mother, my voice cracking with emotion. "They said he might not even make another year at this rate. I hate watching it happen... but what can I do?" I glanced at myself in the mirror behind the bar and saw the tears forming at the corners of my eyes. "The problem is that he needs a chemical crutch to handle life. He's afraid of living without something to blur the edges of reality."

"He's got one good thing on his side, mate. You. And I'm sure you'll get him sorted."

Darren reassurances were well-meaning but I felt empty. Any notion of remedy or cure existing somewhere out there diminished to a far-fetched hope. When Jason can't get enough booze to keep him happy, he uses prescription drugs to top him up, subsidising one with the other. And when he just wants to escape reality completely he uses heroin or crack, whatever's cheapest at the time. He now has drugs to control his hallucinations as well. I looked across at the boy that was my brother, now a man I didn't recognise.

"It's such a difficult one," Darren said, shaking his head in despair. "Until he wants to help himself, you can't do anything but watch. That's awful."

I nodded.

Collecting the drinks, Paul set the glasses in their respective places on our table as if dealing cards whilst Darren and I exchanged questioning glances over the scene at the far corner where my brother had been slouched. In the time it had taken us to get to the bar and back, Jason had become miraculously reanimated. His eyes were full of ardour as he spoke chirpily to an anaemic figure whose complexion blended perfectly with the boarded window. Hemmed in between Richard, Paul and the board, the stranger appeared to have materialised from nowhere, mesmerising my brother with some mysterious narrative we couldn't hear. Jason looked enthralled.

As kids living in Fir Tree Cottage in Sussex, I used to watch my younger brother talk to an unseen stranger with the same focus. Sometimes I could still conjure the image of his face, engrossed yet puzzled as he talked to the invisible person in his bedroom. A person I could never see but that he claimed was there. I remember thinking I must be lacking in some way.

Jason often communicated with his imaginary friend during times of stress, perhaps because he felt the only way he could placate things was by humouring and accepting this imaginary presence. Yet was it also somehow the source of his illness, where it all originated? I suspected part of the answer was lying somewhere amid the rubble of childhood memories.

There was one tangible feeling I do remember about Fir Tree Cottage, which is that what I didn't see I sometimes sensed. Yes, there was a strange, unsettling feeling there. I once doodled a creepy poem in my notebook during a long train journey, contemplating those days of our childhood:

> *What is it you see, when I sit on my bed?*
> *Is it a shadow in your head?*
> *A ghost, a ghoul, the evil dead?*
> *To fathom the conundrums of your mind*
> *would help you heal your restless grind.*

"That's my brother, Marc. He's a great brother!" Jason interrupted my daydream, happily pointing me out as my friends tried to conceal their amusement. "Marc, this is Steve. He's a great mate of mine."

The spectre shook my hand timidly and I succumbed to a tidal wave of compassion for this other sorry creature. It was like shaking the hand of a sick child. Chances are this would be another of Jason's 'friends' that I would at first feel sorry for before he stole Jason's most treasured belongings.

2

PILLOW TALK

It had gone midnight and I'd been asleep on the sofa for over an hour. A small noise woke me. I watched Jason. Kneeling on the floor in front of me, he appeared to be asleep, his flickering eyelids the only evidence of consciousness.

"You okay, Jason?"

There was no response. Was he sleepwalking? He'd done similar strange things before, like the time I'd found him asleep in my garden, draped over the gate. Scrutinising him, I realised that although he was partially comatose he was still trying to erect the thickly padded sun lounger I'd given him to sleep on. I had thought that this would better suit my brother's long frame than the two-seater sofa and hoped he'd finally get some rest. According to him, he'd only had two hours' sleep in the past three days.

I'd stayed up late this Friday night to keep him company and to make sure he went to bed safely without setting fire to the house. The haphazard way he littered ash from the cigarette fluttering in the corner of his mouth always made me anxious.

Now, watching him like this, I was reminded of our childhood adjoined bedrooms in the cottage. I'd regularly sit as a silent voyeur, marvelling at my brother's ability to play endlessly with perpetual concentration and imagination as he dressed his

Action Men and re-equipped them for another epic adventure the next day.

Without acknowledging me, Jason pulled down both folded ends of the sun lounger and they clicked into place. His mouth curled into a smile, sending a further sprinkling of ash floating onto the carpet.

"Use the ashtray, Jason. Please." I slid the dissected Cola can he'd improvised earlier, using the scissors from his Swiss Army knife, across the coffee table. My brother looked hurt. I hated scolding him but I had my kids' welfare to consider.

"Did you know," Jason began muttering semi-incoherently, a cigarette glued to the corner of his lips, "an average person has one thousand four hundred and sixty dreams per year?"

I was too tired to ask what documentary he'd digested this fact from and contemplated whether I should quickly intervene and put the bed up for him myself so I could finally get some sleep. But turning the half-opened lounger on its side, Jason surveyed it intensely with the self-satisfied look of someone who'd finally solved a Rubik's Cube.

"Marc, did you know elephants can sleep standing up?"

"Maybe you have elephant DNA then, Jason. You seem able to make up a sun lounger while in a partial coma." I tried counting the cider cans dotted around the room. He looked up at me with a confused expression.

"I'm not in a coma. Anyway, I'm going to get some sleep now, Marc," he muttered. "And thanks for letting me stay. Thanks for what you do for me. You're a good brother."

"There's no need to thank me so bloody much, Jason."

He snapped the front portion of the lounger into place with a reassuring clunk as his eyelids lost the fight against gravity.

Earlier that afternoon, Jason had phoned me from the local library, already well oiled. An idea had obviously possessed him as he'd walked back home after meeting his key worker, Trisha. She'd been trying to encourage him to do something productive with his once fruitful mind. Trisha was aware that in his earlier life Jason had been a promising artist; he'd told her about the external examiner who'd assessed his work for the Art Foundation course and had even purchased three of his paintings.

With his idea in mind, Jason had approached the young woman sitting at her desk in the library, and asked if she'd look up '1970s priests' on her computer for him. Evidently, she was as confused as Jason because then he'd decided to phone me for more information.

"What was the name of the priest from the seventies who came to the cottage, Marc?" he demanded. When these requests for information possessed my brother, there was always a heated urgency, almost a passion about them.

"Dom Robert Petitpierre," I told him. "Why are you looking him up now?"

A long-hidden memory of Dom Robert strolling across our garden to greet us flashed into my mind. Jason explained he'd been frustrated during his meeting with Trisha as he'd been trying to explain a bit about his past, hoping he'd impress her with the name of the famous priest who'd once visited Fir Tree Cottage. Petitpierre had also written a brief account in his memoirs of the exorcism he performed all those years ago after our builders, preparing the place for us to move in, fled without warning, claiming that 'something' in the cottage wanted them out.

Jason was often obsessed about random childhood recollections, perhaps in an effort to find answers for himself in the process. That particular chapter, though, was an event we rarely discussed even now. It was too off the wall.

Having told the librarian the name of the priest, she soon had a screen full of facts which Jason proceeded to relay down the phone to me.

"Did you know he wrote a book about exorcism for the Church?" he asked.

"Yes, I knew that," I told him.

"And did you know he also exorcised the Astor mansion where Christine Keeler held sex parties?"

"I did. I'll see you tonight, Jason, and we can talk about it then."

As usual I'd had little prior notice from Jason that he was effectively homeless again. So now I had him back until he could find something more permanent. I was always the easiest route to uncomplicated shelter; there would be too many difficult questions if he rocked up at our mother's without notice.

One memorable time I'd ventured into the box room at Mum's house one morning to check up on him at her request. From the waist down his body was draped across the mattress he'd slept on; the rest of him, along with the bedclothes, was on the floor. Studding the carpet were cans of White Star cider, some decorated with cigarette ash and tobacco, one ominously upturned with a syringe protruding from the top.

Downstairs our mother sat in despair, tear tracks on her cheeks. The previous evening, after agreeing to let him stay again, she'd prepared his old bedroom and retired, her heart heavy at the tangible decline of her son. She rightly believed that it was the kindest, if hardest, thing not to allow him to live there as a ravaged, intravenous heroin user. But sometimes she couldn't turn him away. She'd listened to the ranting monologues from his room that evening as they continued into the early hours, searching her mind for a way to help him.

As the morning light slid through her curtains her first thought was of her son's jumbled words about conspiracy theories, chaotic documentary facts and mutterings about something always following him wherever he went. Jason had claimed, ever since his life spiralled downwards in his late teens, that whatever he'd seen when first entering Fir Tree Cottage had followed and tormented him ever since. Somehow he'd made the decision that drugs were the only real solution to his tormented mind.

Still unaware of me in the doorway, my brother woke up and perched on the corner of his defiled mattress, retrieving a cider can from beside his feet, slurring semi-coherently to himself.

"…the loneliest creature on Earth is a whale," he mumbled.

"They can call out for a mate for over two decades… but their voices are so different, other whales never respond."

I wondered whether his regurgitated fact was true. Surely he was the loneliest creature on Earth. I remembered Mum telling me how Jason would cling to her like a spider monkey at his nursery when we first moved to Fir Tree Cottage. She'd have to prise away his gripping fingers in order to leave him there. Sometimes she felt so guilty she'd stay and help out.

Jason reached into the pocket of his grimy sheepskin jacket and pulled out a small pouch of Golden Virginia, cigarette papers and some ominous-looking silver foil. As he unwrapped the small package to check the contents, his memory of the previous night became lucid and painfully real.

"I'm such a fuckup," he said. "I just can't stand my fucking life." Placing the wrap on the table, he started to sob bitterly, his tears dropping from his face and splashing at his feet.

Since then it had been easier for everyone concerned if Jason stayed at mine when he had nowhere else to go. Now I watched him move to the other end of the sun lounger and pull the section flat with another resounding clunk.

"These are good, these loungers, Marc. They're well made. I should have bought one myself years ago." He pulled down the undercarriage legs, turned the bed upright and patted it with a triumphant smile. "That cushion feels well comfortable, Marc. Compared to what I've slept on the last few weeks. Thanks for this. Thanks for what you do for me."

"Jason. Shut up and go to bed please."

Perched on the corner of the sofa I watched him shimmy off his jeans, carefully placing them over the armchair. As usual my heart started to break as I studied him, unable to conceal my dismay. Even the thermal underwear he wore underneath was decrepit. Pulling down the arms of his top, both elbows poked through respective holes.

Another memory of the bedroom at the cottage resurfaced, my brother in pyjamas holding up his Action Man and silently surveying the matted vegetation outside his window. This is what hurts most, the thought of Jason's troubled journey through life since those innocent days of childhood.

"At least the elbows and knees match, eh, Jason?" Humour proved fruitless. He didn't register my remark.

"Did you know the body never adjusts to shift work, Marc?"

"Don't think you're going to have to worry about that anytime soon, Jason."

"Once I'm clean though, Marc, I'm going to be the head of a massive international conglomerate," he mumbled. I couldn't help marvelling, as he now stood swaying unsteadily over the sun lounger, at his miraculous ability to pronounce multi-syllabled words. He held a can up towards his face and tilted it from side to side. "Can't sleep on an empty stomach, Marc."

He knelt down, lifted the bed covers and wriggled himself slowly inside. "Sleep's as important as diet and exercise," Jason educated me.

"You'd better get some then, mate. We'll tackle the diet and exercise regime tomorrow, yeah?"

"Thanks for letting me stay."

I went to leave the room and switched off the light.

"Marc?"

I paused at the door and faced him.

"Do you know an albatross can sleep while it fli—?"

A loud metallic clang interrupted his words as the back of the lounger collapsed, rendering his prostrate body at an absurd angle, feet pointing above the television. He rolled onto the floor.

"Fuck," he declared.

"You didn't pull the legs out properly, Jason."

Vexed, he gritted his teeth and shook his fist at the lounger before yanking the legs into position again with a reassuring thud. Sliding back under the covers, he steadied himself with one foot on the floor. Satisfied that everything was now fully stabilised, he quickly brought his other leg under the covers and lay motionless like a mummy, hardly daring to move. He turned his head cautiously and faced my silhouette in the doorway.

"That's better. Sorry, Marc. Sorry to be a nuisance. Thanks for—"

The bed clanged loudly again as the feet gave way.

The notion of sleep for either of us was becoming a fantasy so I switched the light back on while he tried all over again.

"Sorry. I know I'm a nuisance. Thanks though, thanks for letting me sleep here. Sorry! Did you know that vampire bats sometimes feed on sleeping humans?"

He began rambling an array of random bat facts. It was a good moment to leave him as I knew this way his mind would slowly calm and he'd hopefully sleep for a few hours. That was my earnest hope at least.

In the morning, I found that he'd given up on the lounger and removed all its cushions along with those on the sofa to make a nest on the floor. I brought us both some coffees.

"Do you remember sleeping in that bedroom when we were kids, Marc?" he asked.

I nodded, recalling last night's memory of him standing at the window, staring out into the side garden of the cottage.

"I used to worry about someone clambering onto the lean-to roof and coming into my window," Jason said.

"Who would want to do that?" I said, considering his claims with my usual scepticism. Perhaps this particular memory was just a partial dream. Time passes at the speed of life until childhood events become fragments of fragile memories that make no sense.

"I used to see orbs outside the window at night," he began. "I would look through the eye of my Action Man. Do you remember my Eagle Eye Action Man?" My brother had a toy chest full of Action Man paraphernalia. Along with his tatty blanket comforter, they were always his most trusty pacifiers.

"So, how did the meeting go yesterday with your key worker, Jason?" I asked, once we'd both woken up properly.

"She was alright, but the psychiatrist bloke or social worker or whatever he is was a right wanker." There was venom in his voice. "He was asking me the same fucking questions over and over, didn't even look at me as he asked them. It was like he was reading off of a worksheet."

"What were the questions?"

"What made me want to take drugs in the first place? I answered that question the last time I saw him and the time before that. He doesn't even listen to my answers."

"What did you answer?"

"I told him I just wanted to finally escape everything. I read a book about drugs when I was twelve or thirteen which explained what they all do to you and I thought drugs would be nicer than real life which is why I started using them."

I could understand that this would seem perfectly reasonable to my brother.

"Then he asked me about my mother and family," Jason continued. "I always tell them that I love my mother and my brothers. You're a great brother to me, Marc."

"Enough, Jace." My hand went up to silence him.

"He asked about Dad as well." Jason bit his lip.

"What do you tell them about him?"

"The same thing every time. That he left when I was about five. How difficult is it for them to remember that? I've seen the same guy for months and he asks the same stupid questions. He's not interested enough to remember the fucking answers."

It was a valid and sad observation.

"Maybe you should tell them you believe you're an alien who's been instructed to sample all the different drugs in the world and compile a report on them," I said, trying to lift the mood.

"Come on, they'd think I was a complete loony if I said that," he mumbled, gazing at the television.

I recognised, and not for the first time, how hard this was for Jason, how indifference always hurt him. I tried to imagine being in the same position, feeling vulnerable and having to tell a stranger my fears and problems, then repeat it all again the following week. How many troubled souls faced the same journey as my brother?

"So, did anything good come out of your meeting, Jace?" I pressed him. "There must be something positive surely?"

"No," he snapped in resignation, staring at the screen. "Failed the piss test again. I always fail the piss test. Positive for drugs and alcohol. I don't know why they waste their time."

3

UNWASHED AND
SOMEWHAT DAZED

Jason's key worker had requested that I accompany him to his next meeting. I took the morning off work as he'd become increasingly unreliable at keeping appointments. I didn't know her motives for requesting my presence, but I was still hopeful that after trying to get him help for many years a plan of action was finally unfolding.

There were, though, two likely motives to contemplate. Firstly, that his key worker was inquisitive about the family support my brother had should they finally get him into rehab. Funding was hard-fought for these places and candidates were vetted for likelihood of success. Without support when a client left rehab, they knew that a swift relapse was highly likely.

Less positively, I also suspected that his key worker simply wanted to demonstrate the one-way battle she endured with Jason and why, despite her best efforts, rehab may not work in his case. If he wasn't trying hard enough to help himself, the taxpayers' money would be wasted and another limited resource would be flushed well and truly down the drain.

But if Jason could show commitment, and display convincing willpower that he was taking these first steps on his own, perhaps there was a small chance the council might take that plunge and help him with the rest of the journey.

The imaginary debate continued in my head as I watched my brother drift haphazardly from one side of the pavement to the other on our short walk to the Centre.

It seemed to me, at least, that Jason had been showing genuine signs of wanting to help himself and finally change his life. So the question really being asked of him was, did he have the motivation and ability to help himself? The system wasn't set up to motivate you; you had to meet it halfway. Despite constant protests that he'd 'not had a drink' or 'hadn't touched a thing for a week', which I knew were lies, he had been showing signs of increasing despair with the non-direction of his life. He'd even begun talking about getting clean and getting a job.

Still, I struggled to convince myself there was any possible future for my brother other than premature oblivion.

The Centre was split between two dingy redbrick buildings. The grey windowpanes and their peeling frames gave the impression of dereliction awaiting destruction. Despite this crumbling facility, my brother's key worker had become a source of continuity and stability for him. We were both thankful for her continued efforts. Other care workers had come and gone and Jason would mumble incessantly about them, reeling off the unpronounceable name of yet another psychiatrist or doctor who had left him in the lurch again.

I pushed open the doors and Jason rolled into the Reception and slapped his hands on the desk.

"Hello, darling. Missed me, have you?"

Eyes half open, he made various attempts at a cheeky wink that only resembled an awkward nervous tic. Patches of missed stubble shadowed his face and the nicotine stain on his front tooth hung like an exclamation mark to his unique expression of unkempt abandonment.

"Jason King?" The dour middle-aged women asked, trying to hide her aversion to my brother's obvious reek. Jason straightened abruptly as if about to salute.

"Yeah."

"Can you do me a urine sample please, Jason?"

My brother leered at me. He did this often to defuse his anxiety.

"You don't fancy doing this for me do you, Marc?" He waved the bottle at me with a syrupy laugh, before following the nurse down the hallway. I smiled apologetically to the receptionist and waited to be summoned to Trisha's office.

"Haloperidol, 500 micrograms…"

Jason sniffed hard and wiped his tar-stained fingers onto the back of the prescription receipts he was reading from. Trisha had asked him to bring a list of his current prescription drugs. At the corner of her table, I sat silently like a ghost witness to my brother's despair. In the space of five minutes, his flippancy had collapsed to despondency and I watched his tears pat steadily onto the green prescription paper.

"Diazepam 10 mg… that's to keep me calm," he explained, wiping his eyes. "I can have four of them a day. Temazepam 20 mg. I think that helps me sleep. Citalopram 20 mg. That's for depression. I have one every day. Buprenorphine 2 mg and 400 micrograms… I take them every day… I think that's a heroin substitute. I don't do heroin anymore. And the pericarditis is behind me." It was true that his pericarditis – the swelling of the pericardium, the fluid-filled sac surrounding the heart – was now only a sporadic problem Jason experienced when he drank hard.

Now he gazed at Trisha, hoping for some acknowledgement or approval. Jason had managed to stop himself taking heroin intravenously, undeniably his most notable achievement to date. He'd scored his first hit of heroin when he was only sixteen, and I have always kicked myself for not being aware of this at the time.

Trisha didn't comment.

"I take cocaine… I smoke it but I don't shoot up any more." Jason looked up briefly before letting his head drop like a stone. Perhaps my second guess had been correct: I was there as a witness to hopelessness, as my brother undid himself before us. I feared his last chance to change the trajectory of his life was about to go horribly wrong.

"How much do you use a week?" Trisha asked.

"Three to four hundred pounds or so."

I must have reeled visibly as Jason blurted this out, his voice breaking as he began crying again, his head turning slowly from side to side, his shoulders spasming. Trisha picked up a box of tissues and placed them on his lap.

"How much do you drink a day, Jason?" she asked softly,

"Drink? I've cut down… but about six or eight cans a day or so."

"What of?"

"White Star cider… white cider, the strong stuff."

"The urine test confirms exactly what you've told me, Jason," Trisha tapped the specimen bottle on the table between us. "You're positive for cocaine and alcohol. Thanks for your honesty."

She then asked the question that was spinning around my own head, how he could afford such a big habit. After all, he was on benefits, unemployed and practically homeless, hopping from couch to couch, from squat to squat.

"I've got my means," Jason retorted vitriolically. His legs began bobbing up and down like pistons on an engine. The silence was overwhelming.

"Jason?" Trisha said. "Do you sell yourself for money?"

"No, I fucking don't!" he hissed, spraying spittle onto the table. "I had some money. It was left to me by my grandfather." Stammering, he protested angrily at the suggestion again before finally admitting that he'd now used all of that money on drugs. Now, he hinted, getting drugs on tick was not a problem for him.

"What is it you actually want to achieve, Jason?"

"I want to stop it all," he bellowed, legs dancing nervously, before sobbing into a clump of tissues.

"The drink too?"

"Everything. I just want to be normal." His voice diminished to another pitiful sniffle as he blew fiercely into the tissues.

"Why do you have to use the Haloperidol, Jason?" She

explained that his legs bobbing up and down in coordination with his anxiety was a common side-effect. She understood how socially uncomfortable this spontaneous leg movement must make him feel and she could look at alternatives for him. "But why did the doctor put you on Haloperidol?" she repeated.

"I take it…" he looked at Trisha, his eyes welling again. After a long silence, he finally said, "…because it stops me seeing things."

"What do you see?"

"Things."

"How long has this been going on, Jason?" she asked.

"I can't remember. You'll think it's the drugs and booze but it's not. It even happens when I'm straight. It's been happening all my life. Since I was a kid." Trisha was making a note of this when Jason suddenly played all his cards. "They follow me about. I see things out of nowhere."

He'd always maintained that something had troubled him since he was a child, but it was the first time Trisha had heard this.

As her questioning persisted – what sort of things he saw, if they happened in dreams or when he was awake – I couldn't tell if she wanted to simply understand my brother's condition or confirm her suspicions that he was clearly more unwell than anyone thought. All I could imagine was his inevitable sectioning, the long stretch in a mental hospital, the very last thing that Jason wanted to happen next.

"It was when we lived in this cottage in Sussex. It all started then," he told her, yanking out another clump of tissues.

Trisha encouraged Jason to go on, it was good for him to talk about it, it was necessary if they were to have any chance of understanding the cause of his illness and how best to help him. There always had to be a reason, a natural explanation, for mental illness. Jason himself appeared resigned at this point. It was up to them, he said, the psychiatrists, the key workers and doctors, to decide if he was mad or just sad, because he didn't care anymore. He didn't understand anything about his life.

"You wouldn't believe what I've seen."

With resignation, he began to tell his story, the same one he'd often rolled out to me, as Trisha picked up her pen again and resumed her note-taking.

"I don't think we'd been living in the cottage very long. I woke up because I could hear a voice. It was praying or chanting. I remember it like it was yesterday. Marc's bed was on a different level to mine, up some steps, there was only a banister separating our rooms. When I sat up, I could see someone kneeling beside his bed. It looked like they were praying."

He described this figure as being darker than the darkness that surrounded it, darker than the room and the night. My brother stared blankly at the wall, as if still listening to the sound of the prayers he'd heard and could still see the figure rocking back and forth. Trisha tried to reason with him, asking if perhaps the figure was someone he knew, his father or a friend.

"Not my fucking father,' he replied irritably. "He was long gone by then. It was a no-one, just a figure. It looked like someone but it wasn't."

"What did you feel when you saw this figure?"

"I was shocked. Frightened. So I hid under the bed covers."

I'd always questioned Jason's claims about the supernatural influences on his life. Of course, I knew the history of the cottage and what the builders claimed had happened there, but so did he. So his disturbed mind was more than capable of conjuring wild tales, imaginary or otherwise.

Trisha asked Jason if he'd ever spoken to anyone about it at the time. My brother looked at me. Trisha looked at me. I shrugged. I've always considered myself agnostic, yet it was true to say there were things that never sat right with me when we lived in the cottage. I couldn't decide if I should breezily agree that my brother had mentioned this episode, or admit that I still had a faint memory of being woken one night from a bad dream and hiding under my covers, believing there was a stranger near my bed. Hasn't every kid had more than a few nightmares?

"We were often scared in that place," said Jason. "But we

liked playing outside in the garden, didn't we, Marc?" All I could do was nod and smile at Trisha politely. "It's been going on ever since, though," he continued. "It's followed me around, pretty much wherever I live. I know… you probably think I'm a mad druggie drunk… which I am."

As Trisha asked how often he saw things now and if he ever heard voices, a dreadful wave of vulnerability rushed over his face.

"Yes. I hear voices and see things," he replied with a sarcastic tone, as if to say 'and what the fuck are you going to do about it?'

"We're out of time I'm afraid, Jason," Trisha suddenly announced without looking up from the form she was writing. "Sorry. I know it's hard for you to talk about these things but I am trying to help. I think we should make a referral for you to see our head psychiatrist with me. Would that be okay?"

"Yeah…" his voice breaking, "…whatever."

We walked out of Trisha's office and towards the waiting room. A Hendrix tune was playing on the radio and I watched my brother become immediately intoxicated by the sound. Two strangers stared at him as he declared passionately, "I fucking love this song!"

On the way back to his place I tried to reassure Jason he'd done well, but his horror with himself was tangible. And it worried me that perhaps I hadn't done him justice in the meeting, offering up more myself. I had decided, when I agreed to come, that I would only intercede if absolutely necessary. If the object of this meeting was to provide evidence of my brother's needs, there was indeed nothing more I could have added. He'd done that perfectly.

A story I could perhaps have told drifted back to me as we walked and I tried to piece together its chronology in my head, wondering if it would help Trisha to understand my brother. Somehow, I doubted it, though. It had taken me years to understand him.

One December, Jason had agreed to housesit for our grandparents. Sid knew his grandson, then in his late twenties, could be trusted with the promised perks of two weeks in a warm bed, a copious supply of booze and fifty pounds thrown in for good measure. Any damage or losses would result in non-payment but Jason had readily agreed, being desperate for funds.

One night, my cousin Bret and I stood in the middle of the walled garden outside the house. What at first had been intended as a social visit to check up on Jason was about to descend into a hilarious prank. One we thought would be as entertaining for us as for my brother. Gazing up at the majestic starry sky, I pulled the lapels of my jacket up to protect my face from the bitter chill and blew into my hands.

We knew Jason hadn't noticed us. In the dark just beyond the house lights, we sniggered at our clever plan as we approached the lounge windows with cunning precision, careful not to arouse suspicion, and gazed inside. Jason was sitting with his back partially towards us, captivated by the television. Apart from occasional steady swigs from a large can, he was clearly spellbound by the programme.

"Let's move around to the window behind the TV," I whispered to Bret, and we crept across the lawn and positioned ourselves at the large oculus window behind the TV. With his feet on a low brick wall, Bret peered through and glanced at my brother. He giggled as he jumped down from the wall.

"He's staring right at the window," he said. "Come on, let's do it."

We took out the two ghoulish rubber *Scream* masks left over from Bret's Hallowe'en party, complete with black cloth hoods for added realism. The excitement for that brief moment obliterated my instinctive sense of guilt as my cousin spurred me on, reassuring me that it would be an absolute showstopper we'd be laughing about for ages. And although Jason was going to freak out, he would inevitably see the funny side. We were at the point of no return so I pulled the horror mask over my face.

"Come on, let's do this!"

Bret scrambled onto the back wall again, leaned forwards and pushed his face against the window. I got up next to him and could see that Jason was still on the green leather armchair staring intently at the television. He hadn't seen us yet. We watched the animated light from the television play out on his face, his hand steadily tipping the can to his mouth.

"Tap on the window. He's gonna freak," Bret goaded me and I then started tapping and scraping on the window while Bret groaned like a demon. We stopped and waited for a reaction.

Jason suddenly looked away from the television and stared with shock straight at us. Still composed, he then stood up holding his can before pacing backwards to reassess his perspective of what he could see. Tilting his head from side to side, he stared intensely without horror but with acute curiosity.

"He's just staring. He's not crapping himself at all," Bret said, deflated and disbelieving.

We watched Jason stroll casually back to his chair and open another can. Then he stared back at us again, turned off the television and slowly walked out of the room. We'd long stopped laughing.

"Maybe he didn't see us," Bret whispered.

"He must have," I whispered back. "He couldn't have missed us. No-one could have missed that." A shot of guilt began coursing through me as we hovered in the darkness, trying to work it out.

"Well, if he'd seen us, he'd know it was us. He'd know it was a joke," offered Bret.

"What if he didn't? What if he thought we were for real?" I protested.

"Don't be fucking daft," said Bret. "Quick, I think he's coming out. Hide."

We ran back across the lawn, tore the masks from our faces and launched ourselves into the dense vegetation. We lay there waiting, not daring to speak. After what seemed like an age, there was still no sign of Jason. The silence was thunderous. Eventually

I noticed the light fluctuating again through the oculus window so we clambered out of the bushes and made our way back to the low wall.

Guilt and fear were now surging through me like electricity. I watched my dejected brother in the armchair, staring transfixed by the television again. There was no doubt he had seen the two ghouls in front of him but, evidently, to him this was nothing extraordinary. As the lights strobed across his face and illuminated the redness of his eyes, I clearly saw that Jason was crying.

4

THE GREEN PLACE

When my brother and I saw our new home for the first time, even as children we could tell it had an edgy beauty. Reginald Fairfax Wells was an eccentric sculptor who turned his hand to house-building, creating perfect copies of seventeenth century dwellings between the two World Wars. There were more than fifty of them in this area.

Fir Tree Cottage was dilapidated when our father had recognised it as a Wells Cottage during a trip to Sussex, a few months before he told our mother about it. With a talent for creative vision like Jason, he recognised a property that would complete his self-image as an affluent country gent living among the bohemia of the county. Although he wasn't particularly affluent – and I'm pretty sure he was no gent – our mother recognised his drive and ambition, qualities that seduced her and gave her reason to endure him as the marriage went progressively sour. She agreed to the move with the hope that this green place would be the perfect cauldron to produce the magic potion of family harmony.

Only now do I recognise the traits my brother and father share. Both possess undeniable creativity. Our father had exploited his talent, becoming a commercial artist with some of the top agencies in London, where he wined and dined clients with the gift of the gab. With oils, he could copy the Masters without fault and he could conceptualise an entire advertising campaign.

From an early age, Jason could also visually render his thoughts using different mediums such as crayons, pastels and charcoal. Both shared the ability of being able to conjure something from nothing. Although they shared the same artistic gene, where they differed is that our father possessed little compassion. Their personalities were very different too. Our charming father could entertain a crowd but Jason was skilled at inventing solitary games. He'd invent names and characters during our playtime as easily as Leo, our father, could spin a yarn and have friends in stitches.

Jason was acutely sensitive to his environment, quick to become unnerved when the atmosphere turned sour. He was attuned to moods and atmosphere even during his deepest moments of apparent indifference. Unaware of my own concerns it wasn't unusual, while engrossed in a TV programme, for him to ask suddenly, "Are you alright?" before returning to his own thoughts.

Despite their differences, Dad was the centre of Jason's universe. All I remember, however, was an indifferent stranger who was hardly there whilst my brother was acutely aware of a Dad-shaped hole in his life.

When it came to Fir Tree Cottage, our father may have felt he was buying a work of art as well as a quaint country residence. On the other hand, the team of three builders employed to renovate it saw it as a welcome meal ticket, since making a living was proving tough at the time.

To live and work within the walls was the only profitable way to execute the job and their brief was simply to make the place habitable. They would also create another reception room from the adjoining garage with an entrance from the lounge, and the larger bedroom needed to be made into three rooms for the children.

Even as they began the work, our mother told me later, one of the builders had stared up at the cloud reflections in the leaded windowpanes of the cottage feeling inexplicable dread, already sensing that 'something else' was inside the building with them.

Meanwhile, Mum could sense our anxiety about leaving the house we'd lived in for a few years, our unease about starting this new stage of our lives in the countryside. Despite the obvious stress between our parents, this house felt a lot like a home, dependable and familiar, and we had friends nearby.

As we waited to leave, I felt sick with emotion yet adamant my brother shouldn't pick up on my angst. I was his source of stability. Jason endured his emotions silently. He would never whinge or moan if he felt agitated, he was usually too preoccupied with our mother's troubles. Attuned to his feelings, I was painfully aware that another move wasn't going to be easy for him.

While the builders made the cottage ready for us, we would be living at our grandfather's weekend retreat for a few weeks, a bungalow situated just over two desolate miles from Fir Tree Cottage. I found the idea of moving somewhere before you could move somewhere else an impossible concept to grasp, but four year-old Jason needed me to explain things he didn't understand immediately. This was my primary concern since he liked my explanations to be thorough and accompanied with numerous reassurances.

Our mother explained that our grandparents would pick up me, Jason and our baby brother Sean, and take us to their bungalow while she finished cleaning the house and packing up. Then our father would return home and they'd be coming straight away to join us. Leaving Mum behind became another hurdle for Jason.

Grandfather Sid came across as the definitive rough diamond. He was unable to read or write until his early twenties and had had a tough upbringing in London. Sid's mother had died when he was twenty-one and he'd looked after his younger brother and sister on his own. Mum made a point of highlighting his humble beginnings by telling us how he used to get his shoes from the dump.

As we arrived we looked with amazement at the idyllic old bungalow, its three chimneystacks protruding from several unevenly tiled roofs. With only three neighbouring buildings visible, it was obvious the surrounding area was sparsely populated. No friends to play with. Jason clutched the back of my jumper as we anxiously followed our grandfather from the car.

"It looked like a castle when we went through the farm gate into the front garden," Jason reminisced when we talked years later, still clearly remembering his initial impressions. "There was another iron gate like a portcullis opening onto a tiny courtyard before those massive oak castle doors. I was frightened when I first saw them." There were two yellow-tinted windows with bulging oculus panes above the doors, making the place even more spellbinding. "Remember that giant key for the lock, Marc?"

"You wouldn't let go of me, Jason," I remembered. "We must have looked like conjoined twins in our matching jumpers."

"That jumper was as itchy as fuck. I hated it."

Grandfather Sid gradually became less of a harsh stranger and enjoyed sharing this time with us. Jason and I would listen to his playful banter, mesmerised by the heavy gold identity bracelet dancing on his wrist. But although our grandparents tried everything to make us feel at ease, Jason's timidity rendered him monosyllabic. I excused his awkwardness by saying he was just sad about leaving his friends. Eventually, though, our grandmother interceded using her infamous long red nails to gently stroke the back of Jason's hand.

The interior of the bungalow was enthralling. Every square foot of the black ceiling beams and walls in the lounge was festooned with assorted antique horse tack and weaponry such as muskets and shotguns, daggers and Ghurkha knives. Dividing this room from the dining area was the large stone surround of an open fireplace. Two sizeable mantelpieces protruded from each side both littered with curios.

"I couldn't wait to play with the spears and daggers." Childlike, Jason looked as if he'd entered the cottage for the first time again.

Our awkwardness subsided with each new discovery. Investigating the far end of the bungalow we found a large cupboard contained Sid's two shotguns sheathed in canvas gun slips. Two leather cartridge belts swung from a hook inside the door. Our grandmother instructed us sternly not to go into this cupboard because it was where 'Grandad keeps his grown-up toys that aren't for children.' So naturally we earmarked it for later scrutiny since, for children, saying no is as good as an invitation. Despite Jason's anxieties, danger equalled excitement, a fact that's never changed.

"I didn't like that bathroom at the end." Jason suddenly looked uncomfortable with his memories. Although it was cold and unkempt, this room hadn't bothered me despite the peculiar layout, with the toilet in a separate small room. "It was like a fridge inside and the branches outside used to scrape against the windows." Jason's recollections have always consisted of feelings.

As bedtime approached on that first day, my brother's apprehension returned. The countryside was pitch-dark by six o'clock and there was no sign of our parents. We began to fear that we'd be spending our childhood with these two old people, the one with the gold teeth and bracelet and the other with the big red talons. This was, after all, a land where no children existed and the world went black around teatime.

When the front doors clunked open and our mother and father appeared, Jason's relief was tangible. Mum sat on our bed and promised that the following day we'd be going to see our forever home. We went to sleep knowing this new land was going to be an adventure, but we couldn't decide whether it would be a good one or not.

Waking with high anticipation the following morning, we discovered that a thick gloomy mist had enveloped our surroundings. With everyone else still asleep, Jason and I stepped outside and opened the gate to find the quiet lane unrecognisable. The land we'd first set eyes on the previous afternoon was now invisible. The neighbours' roofs and the large barns in the distance crowned by the South Downs had vanished. The trees and dense hedgerow flanking the lane were drained of colour and form. The world stopped just beyond the metal gate to the field opposite, meaning we had barely fifteen yards' visibility. We wondered where all the hills had gone and why all the trees had turned to stone.

A couple of miles away across the lonely fields and winding lanes, according to Mum's later account, one of the builders had also woken early to the mist. Peter, the foreman, and his two fellow builders had now spent nearly a week within the walls of Fir Tree Cottage, but Peter's experiences there had begun spinning his world upside-down. His initial uneasy feeling that something else inhabited the cottage had gained momentum.

During the night he'd heard a voice at random times. Why didn't anyone else hear it? There were inexplicable knocks and bangs from below his room and he was certain that at some point during the early hours he'd been woken by a loud whistle. Peter came to the uncomfortable conclusion that, indeed, there was something else in the cottage.

Of course, we were oblivious to all this at the time. Later that first morning, with Sean sandwiched between Jason and myself, Mum snaked the car through the narrow roads and hollows the mile and a half to the nearby village. The grey-knotted hedgerows towering above the lonely road were intimidating until at last The Queen's Head marked our arrival to the village, the church spire peering above the few small cottages.

The Mini Traveller bucked and crunched along the uneven stones of the country lane like an impromptu fairground ride that would become a familiar sound. Other antiquated cottages haphazardly flanking the lane intrigued us, each shrouded behind high fences or hedges, perfectly manicured and testimony to the loving attention of their retired owners.

Our mother looked in the rear-view mirror and smiled at our expectant faces. Stopping at the end of the drive, she announced, "This is going to be our forever home soon." It was our first glimpse of Fir Tree Cottage and Jason's initial impressions were telling.

"The cottage looked like a sad old lady when I first saw it. I knew I didn't want to move there."

"Why a sad old lady, Jace?"

"The thatched roof was like a droopy sun hat and those two eyelid windows upstairs looked sad, like it was looking down on us."

I also felt something that has never left me about the cottage, a sense of both beauty and sadness. The beauty was most evident in the tranquility of the garden and the birdsong in the trees. We immediately earmarked the large fir tree in the middle of the front garden for a later climbing adventure. Mum promised that once we'd looked around the cottage we could explore the garden for as long as we liked. This filled us with excitement since outside freedom always beat indoor confinement any day of the week.

We followed Mum up the steps to the front patio.

"There was a man filling a crusty cement mixer watching us. I remember him like yesterday," Jason said.

Mum introduced Peter. He was quiet and contemplative with kindness in his eyes. Tired and dirty, Peter attempted to relax Jason by making a fuss of him as he stood staring, hesitant and motionless. Lifting the latch to the front door, Mum led us through the porch into the lounge, still undecorated, bare and empty. The stained and tired floorboards added to the look of abandonment. It was freezing cold and the feeling of dejection returned with a vengeance. Jason took hold of our mother's hand for reassurance.

There was no homeliness, just unadorned brickwork, tools in wraps and boxes strewn across the floorboards. Piles of building materials were stacked disjointedly and rubble lay in heaps in the middle of the lounge waiting to be cleared out. To the right of the porch entrance was a large fireplace with a seasoned oak surround and mantle. From a large man-shaped hole in the wall to the left of this we heard voices and the scraping sounds of shovels on concrete.

I approached and stared through the gap to see the dark void of another room beyond, intimidating and scary. Impatient to find a room with homeliness, I poked my head through and noticed two other builders smiling up at me, a short ladder leading down to what was once an adjoining garage. I turned to Jason to share my discovery of this secret room and its occupants and saw him standing frozen by the porch door.

"There was an old man standing by the fireplace as soon as we walked through the door," Jason still insisted decades later. It didn't matter whether or not he was sober, the story was always the same. "I can still see him as clear as day." He admits that he couldn't see the old man's face lucidly, which has always led me to counter how he could he tell it was an old man. Then he told me randomly one day, "There was someone else. I think they were female." Frowning, he looked towards the heavens as if for some sign of affirmation. "I went back downstairs after seeing the bedrooms and looked at the fireplace again. The figures were gone but instead I saw half a dozen orbs of light bobbing inside the mouth of the fireplace."

I would usually turn off at this point. Yet despite his years of mental and physical erosion, his first impression of the figure in the cottage has never diminished and clearly remains an enigma for him. Sometimes I will point out to him that, as a multi-addict, he couldn't expect to have his claims of unearthly visitors to be treated with credibility.

"If I took that lot every day," I remember saying, nodding at the prescription drugs in his kitchen cupboard, "I'd be seeing ghosts too."

"You know I'm not lying, Marc," he would always plead, looking lost and wounded, making me feel guilty for reminding him what an outcast he'd become over the years.

On our first exploration of the cottage, with its worn-out kitchen and bare floorboards, it appeared to be on the derelict side of basic. The only redeeming feature was the leaded front window affording a wonderful view of the front garden and that fine fir tree we couldn't wait to climb.

"That back kitchen window used to freak me out, though," Jason reminisced. "There were no curtains and I used to think I was being watched at night." Jason stared at the scene in his head. At night with the bare bulbs illuminating indoors, the windows were definitely black as coal.

Between the lounge and kitchen were wooden doors leading to the stairs. With morbid curiosity we ventured further, still hoping the remainder of the cottage would conjure some hope of future happiness. The stairway was dark and creaked with every step as we accompanied the three builders onto the top landing where we were greeted with more bare floorboards and unfinished walls. Peter switched on another inadequate solitary lightbulb.

The builders were a bit older than my parents, perhaps in their mid-thirties, and Peter was overshadowed by his more exuberant colleagues. Their attempts to inject optimism for the renovations faltered immediately when they opened the door to the tiny bathroom where the drab avocado suite looked only fit for the skip. Mum looked unhappy.

"I appreciate it's all a bit crap in here," one of them spoke up. "Your husband doesn't want us to touch the bathroom for the moment. The rest of the place just needs a tidy up for now. A few doors and partitions and you can move in. The whole place was so full of crap."

The other builder ushered us across the landing to the master bedroom on the left. Opening the door, we noticed straight away the double aspect windows providing excellent vantage points to glimpse inside the mysterious fir tree as well as overlooking the back garden.

"Last but not least..." The builder walked back across the landing, flicked the latch to the door opposite and announced,

"The boys' rooms."

Peter's two colleagues beckoned us through. At first the room possessed some vague hope of becoming homely, with a central partition dividing it and a few small steps leading down to a lower floor. In short, our bedrooms were one room dissected, with one half lower by about four feet. A double window peeped from under the thatched roof, which I recognised as a perfect position to spy on both sides of the front garden. Realising the command it gave me over my younger siblings, Mum told me it would be mine.

While I experienced a wave of normality, Jason looked increasingly uneasy. From his lower bedroom, he looked up at the open gap into mine. One of the builders quickly reassured us they'd be erecting a banister across the gap to make it safe but this would still be unobtrusive and allow us to feel we shared one room together.

Peter then watched Mum anxiously as his colleague approached a small cupboard beside the steps. The doors had perfectly spaced holes drilled along the top and bottom giving the impression of a giant kennel or hutch. Screeching the door open we felt the cold chill beyond as he padded inside to locate the switch, presenting us with a room lit by a solitary bulb accompanied by emptiness and neglect. The source of the cold was evident, a large black hole in the plaster-boarded ceiling, yawning into the abyss of the roof.

One of the builders began explaining apologetically that they'd been instructed by Leo to make this space a third bedroom. Everyone looked at Sean perched precariously on my mother's hip. Peter reassured Mum that they would make sure the room was cosy and clean by the time they'd finished, as she tried hard to conceal her dismay. Jason gazed silently into the nebulous space beyond.

"I hated that cupboard they decorated for Sean. It opened into my room," Jason said with dismay.

Mum coaxed us quickly downstairs. We were already deflated about this forever home so she led us out onto the patio, encouraging us to go and explore the garden. Beyond the mossy wooden fence of the garden boundary lay another intriguing wilderness but our first stop was the pond, disregarding our mother's warning to keep away from it.

"I thought it was a swimming pool at first," Jason remembered and certainly, due to its exaggerated proportions, it would have presented that indelible image to a four year-old. Concerned for our safety, Mum's first request to our father had been to have the pond removed. Evidently, despite her protests, this was low down on the to-do list for the builders. We stood on the edge and gazed into the inky black water watching the reflections and dead leaves floating below the surface like fish illuminated by the sun through the parting clouds. Jason, transfixed, needed coaxing from his daydreams.

Racing each other up and down the slope beyond the pond we then realised we were missing out on another adventure. Our father, Leo, had been working at the cottage and had referred on several occasions to his 'studio'. We ran back towards the cottage. On the right was a garage lean-to with a clear corrugated plastic roof, decorated by tree debris and bird shit. To the left stood a posh shed with two ample windows at the front.

What my father did for work intrigued us since we didn't understand what a commercial artist was despite Mum's explanations, especially as she would often mutter despondently that our father was generally more of a piss artist than a commercial one.

The studio was unlocked and inside was a draughtsman's table directly in front of the window, with drawings and plans strewn all over a small table next to it. The place was evidence of our father's secret life. I seem to remember an empty bottle of wine on the table with two glasses and the smell of cologne. We rummaged inside like forensic detectives looking for further clues about Dad, exciting Jason's sense of intrigue and adventure.

"Remember that sex book the old man had in his office drawer, Marc?"

I laughed, recalling how shocked we both were by its discovery. Jason studied the cover with revulsion and confusion. On the black leatherette cover was a line drawing of an exotic couple salaciously entwined. Opening the pages, we gawped at the enlarged line drawings of genitalia, the unfeasible dexterity of the circus-like poses shared between a couple clearly enjoying sex.

I knew what to do with it. He followed as I marched towards the garden fence and propelled it into the dead ferns and fallen branches, hoping it would never be seen again. I remembered my satisfaction, believing it would provide much needed punishment for our father. Jason watched quizzically as I repeated a phrase I'd heard our mother use.

"Dad's a sex maniac, Jason!" I announced, placing my hand reassuringly on my brother's shoulder. We looked at each other perplexed.

"That garden was mysterious. Remember the steep crawl path leading to the back garden behind the lean-to and big green oil tank? And there was a little thatched outhouse surrounded by steep banks we'd climb to get onto the roof and spy on the lane. Remember?" Jason grinned.

I liked doing this memory game with him. It was a curious bleak winter landscape we'd been thrust into which magically reanimated with greenery and colour in the springtime. By the time our mother had finished talking to the builders and yelled our names from the patio, we had a fair idea of what we were in for at Fir Tree Cottage.

"I think we rated the cottage five out of ten just because of the garden," Jason chuckled.

The builders' evening routine didn't vary. They'd work until late, then eat, perhaps enjoy a beer or cheap bottle of wine, simple pleasures to push the working day aside. The pub was unaffordable despite, Peter said later, finding the cottage oppressive. His colleagues fell easily into general bonhomie at the end of the day, whilst Peter felt envious that they could relax as he tried to conceal his unease, contemplating the night-time loneliness ahead. Once it was dark he'd avoid looking through the windows into the blackness, the inside felt dark enough.

He continued to wrestle with his sanity. Knowing he'd soon be alone in his room above the kitchen, he'd try to prolong the conversation, delay the inevitable, but he was tired from all the previous nights. He'd read in his room, but even that usually failed to bring on sleep. He would often endure the early hours trying to rationalise the otherworldly noises he tried desperately not to hear.

While his colleagues slept oblivious in the adjoined room across the landing, he would be startled by random words or obnoxious whistles. Why don't they wake, why was he alone cursed by these disturbances? He'd try and find acceptable excuses for the noises, like cutlery clanking in the kitchen sink, knocks and scrapes coming from other places he couldn't pinpoint. He tried ignoring everything and thinking about home.

One evening he wasn't the only one. Their banter around the kitchen table stopped as a single hammer blow thundered onto the floorboards above. A while later, they'd heard a door or window closing from somewhere distant they couldn't locate. Silently, Peter's colleagues had looked at him for explanation.

But what could he say to them? He couldn't tell them about all the other things he sensed and sometimes saw. They'd think he was mad, a man becoming undone. How could he tell them such peculiarities were plaguing his life and how he already suspected that something paranormal was playing out within the cottage?

He definitely couldn't contemplate telling them that, on the first day they'd stood discussing how to fill in the pond, he'd seen something emerge from the dark water.

5

NEVER GOING BACK AGAIN

It was a weekday morning and the start of another day of work for the builders. The men felt weary, particularly Peter after enduring another restless night. That morning, lying in his room above the kitchen, he tried to comprehend the previous night's creaks and inexplicable noises. Then he got up as usual and peered out of the window across the garden, preparing to face another day.

All we know is that at some point soon after starting work that morning, Peter walked up the stairs as though compelled by a force he didn't understand. He entered the bathroom and was greeted by more than just the drab avocado suite and the dripping basin tap with crusty limescale.

Something within the wooden-framed mirror on the wall startled him as he stared at it. Suddenly the familiar bathroom he thought he was standing in disappeared and instead he found himself in an entirely different place. Where once a tiny window provided minimal light there was only darkness and, somewhere within the room's vague margins, Peter quickly became aware that someone was staring back at him. From downstairs, Peter's colleagues heard shouts of terror. Inside the bathroom, Peter tried moving but his feet felt leaden. The figure within the mirror, its eyes wild, bellowed with fury and a disembodied voice screamed repeatedly at him to get out.

The shock of hearing Peter's shouts could only have been increased by seeing him thundering down the staircase, terrified. He fled the cottage, racing across the front garden and out through the gate into the lane. His traumatised colleagues made the immediate decision to vacate the place too, taking only the keys for the van. Tyres screeching, they escaped through the front gates onto the driveway, following Peter. Then they drove to the bungalow to explain to my father why they would never again set foot inside Fir Tree Cottage.

Mum had put the breakfast washing-up on the drainer and was about to start the drying when she heard the van pull up outside. Shadows loomed in the front door windows and the door handle thudded urgently several times. She couldn't imagine what could be so important at this time of the morning; with no passing traffic, normally the only disturbances were the occasional cawing crows gliding over the fields.

She greeted the builders' unexpected appearance with surprise as first one of them fumbled with an explanation for their visit and then another asked to speak to her husband. As usual, she had no idea where he was. She took the men into the lounge, expecting the worst; whatever was happening, she was going to have to face it on her own as always.

Mum told me later that she checked on Sean, still sleeping in her bedroom, and made sure that Jason and I were occupied. Then she took a chair and sat opposite the men huddled together on the Chesterfield with shell-shocked expressions on their faces. Peter was the spokesman, although he appeared bewildered and was stumbling over his words as he apologised for disturbing her routine. As he couldn't speak to her husband, he'd have to say it to her, though he looked relieved to be doing so.

Mum couldn't believe what she was hearing. Peter was clear in stating firmly that they'd not be going back to finish the work at the cottage. They'd left for good. They apologised profusely for this inconvenience but assured her that a large proportion of the work had been completed. Mum was more than a little perplexed: they were leaving without full payment and without their tools or any of their belongings. Studying them, they appeared liberated rather than dejected. Clearly, they felt that this crazy action was their only option in the circumstances.

My mother was dumbfounded so one of the other men explained that after they'd driven away from the cottage they'd eventually found Peter somewhere within the knot of surrounding lanes, still obviously terrified.

"But what was it that scared you?" she asked Peter.

Taking a deep breath and with eyes wide, he described the alien room inside the mirror and the figure that ordered him from the cottage. Whatever it was, it had been adamant about him leaving, screaming at them to leave the place for good and not go back.

Even that wasn't the last of it.

Peter's colleague explained that when they'd found him, frightened and confused, they'd all agreed to find my father and explain their decision to leave. Then as they switched back through several lanes and side roads, they found themselves back at the entrance of the cottage. They'd set off again, this time taking a different route as they tried to get their bearings and calm down. But there was a just a familiar rumble as the van coasted to a halt and they realised that somehow they had again come full circle and were outside the cottage gates. This happened a third time before they finally located smooth, familiar tarmac and made their way to the bungalow.

Mum was now the mediator, trying to weigh up this strange tale rationally since the formerly laidback builders were displaying signs of lunacy. Was hysteria to blame, the men becoming so wired by the shock of seeing Peter in that state that they'd become disorientated themselves?

Yet her intuition was that they were telling the truth, and she believed them. She was reminded of how our new puppy, Brutus, had behaved on the few occasions she'd visited the cottage unannounced in search of our father. Brutus had become restless, inside the cottage he'd whine and pant and only settled when outside on the patio.

"Hasn't your husband told you about what's been going on at all?" one of the builders asked Mum.

She found it painful to be reminded how little she knew of her husband's other life, his unexplained absences when he was never where he said he would be. Staring at them blankly, she shook her head feeling the onset of panic.

"So this is not the first time... something's happened?" she asked.

Needing to clear her mind, she went to the kitchen, where Brutus was sleeping peacefully, and made tea for them all before settling back down in the lounge. Peter composed himself and then began his account.

They'd commenced work in earnest despite finding it awkward adjusting to their unfamiliar new working environment. The absence of urban noise and the sedate pace felt alien. But they'd kept busy and productive, cracking on with the renovation schedule, grateful for having a lucrative job that might last a month or more. After several days working inside the cottage, they all agreed they could do with a break and decided on The Five Bells, half a mile down the road. Peter especially felt fatigued by the strangely melancholy atmosphere that had set in.

In this area the nights descend quickly during winter. The birdsong disappears in the complete darkness and the peeping lights of neighbouring cottages were the only signs of life. So The Five Bells was a welcome respite. They were pleased to be greeted by friendly, happy drinkers rather than suspicious locals and a sense of normality returned. They decided for the time being they'd adopt the pub as their new local, with its cosy atmosphere and curling cigarette smoke in sharp contrast to the bleakness of the cold, gloomy cottage.

When it was getting late they decided to leave. Peter assured Mum they'd only had a few pints that evening with their meal, so they were more or less sober. Outside in the brisk chill of the still night air they were all in happier spirits as they climbed into the van and rumbled back towards the cottage. Peter had begun to consider the prospect of another uneasy night but tried to put the thought out of his mind as he drove the van slowly up the driveway. Then suddenly one of the men urged him to stop, putting a hand firmly on his shoulder.

Within the shaft of the headlights' beam, a figure stood motionless in the dusty vapour of light mist against the whitewashed wall of the lean-to. The trespasser seemed to be standing in a confrontational, brazen manner, unflinching and staring directly back at them. Curiously, according to all three, his features couldn't be made out in the dazzle of the beam yet they assumed him to be old by the odd slant of his body.

Two of the men decided to confront the man, their bravado perhaps fuelled a little by alcohol, and they jumped out of the van. They shouted at the trespasser, asking why he was there and what he wanted, assuring him that if he had no good reason he'd be forcibly ejected from the grounds. They were greeted with a stony silence and the same unflinching stance.

As they marched towards the trespasser he leered at them before shifting seamlessly like mist behind the lean-to. So it was now a chase. They shouted at Peter to get out of the van and help cut the man off when he emerged around the other side. Peter said he'd felt nervous, cemented to the driving seat. How could he tell his mates that he suspected he'd seen this trespasser before, on that first day when they were wondering how best to fill in the pond? At the time, he hadn't been entirely sure what he'd seen but his mind had rationalised it was a figure that had risen up from the pond. But he remembered, as he'd turned away to walk back to the patio, how it lingered momentarily before disappearing around the back of the cottage.

Peter finally stepped out of the van into the blackness. Walking cautiously across the lawn to one side he heard the angry shouts of his colleagues, the trampling of undergrowth and snapping of twigs piercing the silence of the garden. He crept around the back of the cottage trying to adjust his vision as he deliberated what to do should the figure confront him.

The other men called again for Peter's help, believing they were closing in on the trespasser, so he clambered up the bank to the back of the outhouse. Somehow everything appeared different to what he remembered, the bank much steeper and his progress hindered by a labyrinth of dense undergrowth and dry, sharp tree branches forming an impregnable barrier. Surely this hadn't been there before? The men shouted again, sounding vexed, so Peter crawled through the undergrowth, the branches scratching his face and hands.

Finally he found them. Between them they'd covered the entire circumference of the rear garden but the trespasser had vanished. In the stillness, Peter considered whether to share his gut instinct that perhaps they'd given chase to something other than a man – but what could he say it was?

Shivering in the middle of the back garden, they decided to retrace their steps, battling again with the branches and brambles. Peter followed in thoughtful silence, listening to his cursing workmates. Back on the driveway again, bathed in the vapour of the headlights, Peter stared at the van. He knew perfectly well that he'd turned the engine off before leaving it, yet the engine was now running.

Deciding the trespasser was long gone they entered the cottage apprehensively. They wondered whether perhaps it was a tramp who sometimes lived within the grounds since he clearly had a far better knowledge of the garden than they did. If so, the visitor might even consider them to be the trespassers.

Mum was listening carefully while trying to control her rising anxiety. Their account sounded more like something you'd read in a novel and this was not the new life she was hoping to begin with her children. And where the hell was her husband? She needed to find a rational explanation. If this was a tramp, he could be reasoned with.

But then Peter explained that this was only the start of the strangeness. The following morning they had relived the previous night's experience while looking out across the garden. The most puzzling aspect of it all wasn't so much the disappearance of the stranger but the barrier of sharp undergrowth they'd encountered. They looked again at the scratches and puncture marks on their hands, faces and necks; there was clearly no such vegetation in the garden, only wasted coppice and grey tree branches, the whole area lifeless with the onset of winter. They walked out to inspect it, retracing the previous night's steps and walking a full circumference confirming that there was no blockade of spiky branches. Peter walked easily up the shallow bank behind the outhouse, realising that even the earth had conspired against them.

At night, Peter would busy himself constructing a fire, tightening twists of old newspaper and placing them in the hearth as he listened to his mates' theories again. He had a feeling they were partly correct, the visitor felt entitled to the cottage and they were the trespassers. Placing a mound of kindling on top of the newspaper he'd flick a match, knowing he wouldn't sleep again tonight. Maybe it was his duty to stay awake, like a night-watchman.

My mother says that a definite chill ran down her back when Peter began to detail the strange noises he heard. On the very first night he'd twice heard a loud wolf whistle, like a deliberate taunt, from somewhere he couldn't fathom within the cottage. It was a desperate situation for him, being unable to explain anything to the others even though they were friends, so at first he endured these abnormalities alone. He admitted that he'd been dogged most of his life with some sort of ability to perceive paranormal things. He'd always feared people would think him mad if he spoke about it.

"Are you talking about... ghosts?" Mum asked him. He shrugged, saying he didn't really understand what it was all about.

On other nights, some of the spoken sounds he heard were repeated, jumbled words, names and phrases that all three of the men had previously spoken – and Peter heard them in their individual voices. Sometimes, even the other men had also heard these repeated words during the day, trying to laugh it off as the work of 'Fred the ventriloquist'.

Only the fire at night in the cottage, with its warmth and light, kept the cold and malevolence at bay. With the logs crackling in the grate, sending licking flames into the blackness of the chimney, they would begin to relax. The men clutched the idea that perhaps after all there was some natural explanation to be found for all the strangeness.

Then one night, just as they drained the last of their tea from their cups, a loud bang shook the windows. The shock wave echoed throughout the cottage and the diamond panes downstairs shuddered within their lattice frames. The sound came from the back door of the kitchen. Inside the dimly lit kitchen one of the men tried opening the door, tugging hard on the handle but finding it resolutely stuck. It was evident the door couldn't have slammed in the way they'd heard. They stared at the window into the charcoal blackness with a feeling they were being observed.

Just then the air around them shifted in a powerful gust. They stared behind them in shock at the swaying lounge door. Back inside the lounge they expected to feel warmth, hear the crackle of the burning logs, but instead the hearth was black, the fire extinguished as if it had never been lit.

Mum told me that at this point her throat had felt dry and the palms of her hands were moist with anxiety, but when she reached for her cup the tea had gone cold. Going into the kitchen to make fresh drinks, she was reminded of an unexplained incident with a kettle at the cottage one afternoon. She'd been asked to take a replacement kettle to the cottage for the builders since the old one had broken, much to the annoyance of our father who was becoming impatient with the various hold-ups occurring. She walked inside and shouted a greeting before going into the kitchen and filling the kettle. Only then did she notice that it didn't have a plug fitted.

She went to find one of the builders and Peter was in the old garage adjoined to the lounge. They began a conversation and soon the other two men joined them, bringing in cups of tea and coffee. Mum thought nothing of it until she remembered she had to collect us from our grandparents and had left the car keys on the kitchen drainer. As she picked them up she saw that the kettle still had no plug; she hadn't told the men about fitting one.

She'd tried to rationalise this. Had one of them had fixed a plug and then for some unexplained reason taken it off again? Even so, in the time it took for the men to come downstairs, go to the kitchen and then come to the garage, it would have been an impossible to fit a plug and make hot drinks. Moreover, the hob was also not working so there was no other way to boil water.

With a hundred things on her mind she'd had no time to question the builders before leaving and the puzzle hung in her head like a question mark. Returning to the lounge, she told the dazed builders her story and they assured her they'd not bought a replacement kettle.

The men agreed that the regular inexplicable mayhem occurring could no longer be considered as mischievous pranks played on each other. Any affection they'd harboured previously for 'the ventriloquist' was gone and it was clear they felt foolish for considering the events as anything but paranormal for so long.

One of the men described the negative effects they'd been having. For example, one afternoon he'd gone upstairs to continue work and found his tools missing. He remembered leaving them in a canvas wrap on the floor and was meticulously about tidiness. But these disappearances were becoming regular occurrences and led to accusations between them about practical jokes becoming tiresome. The men regularly found themselves becoming uncharacteristically aggressive and angry with each another. They confessed they'd been at the point, during these squabbles, of lashing out with frustration.

But during these last few weeks, they didn't react if their tools weren't where they left them or a paintbrush was no longer in a pot but on the floor of another room. Once they'd found sheets of plasterboard previously leaning carefully against a wall had thundered down onto the floorboards. At these moments they'd group together and wait, knowing that they'd soon hear a thump from upstairs, an unrepentant whistle or shout, their own names being called. Whenever they investigated shouts or whistles, they'd hear them repeated from another room they couldn't place. If one man was in a room and heard his name shouted, he no longer questioned his mates. They came to accept that it was an entity toying with them and, by accepting it, they began doubting their own sanity.

As an adult, I listened to Mum's account of that extraordinary conversation like an agnostic listening to a sermon. I've always sought alternative explanations. Even though I'd lived there as a child and have Jason's descriptions of his own experiences, and even though I've since read about the exorcism carried out later by Dom Robert Petitpierre at the cottage, I clung to my scepticism. Yet the fact I found most difficult to rationalise was how grown men could be prepared to sacrifice their livelihoods so readily. Perhaps that was better proof of something other than simply misplaced tools or shifting shadows.

The men had sat in awkward silence after finishing their account until at last Peter smiled at Mum and advised her to 'have the place looked at' before moving in. They thanked Mum for listening and got up to leave, asking her to apologise on their behalf to Leo. They kept apologising as they left, like naughty children admitting to an offence they didn't understand.

After the van had left, Mum smoked a couple of Silk Cuts thinking about what she could do. This was beyond her understanding. She wrestled with the problem all day until finally, late in the evening, she walked into the hallway, opened the telephone directory and dialled the number listed for the Reverend Jones.

Years later, after renewing contact with our father, I approached the subject of the cottage warily. It was obvious from his expression I'd inherited my agnostic outlook from him. He shook his head ruefully at the time it had taken to renovate the cottage.

"There was one thing that I've never been able to explain, though," he began, still questioning the reality.

On every occasion the builders had come to him complaining about abnormal occurrences, he'd dismissed their stories as nonsense. He couldn't believe these were the self-same men he'd hired for the task; their easy-going nature had become unhinged and couldn't fathom their change of attitude. It was mostly Peter who'd tried his patience. He treated everything he was told as farcical, fictitious even, assuming their motive was simply to buy more time on the job and make more money. He was neither empathetic to their feelings nor open to the possibility of another reason for the decline in their moods.

He'd walked in on Peter one afternoon and found him kneeling down hammering the floorboards. After shouting at him several times, Peter jumped to his feet startled, appearing troubled and uncertain. They had a short conversation about the progress of the job, during which Peter brought up again the subject of strange happenings. It was becoming an irritatingly regular occurrence and Leo was losing patience. He dismissed Peter's claims, assuming his tired and dishevelled appearance was the result of him overdoing it at The Five Bells. He felt he no longer knew Peter and began to believe he'd chosen the wrong men to complete the work. Aggravated, he wondered how much more of this negativity and inertia he could endure.

Leaving Peter to carry on, Leo had gone upstairs to check on the rest of the builders. When he reached the landing he stood in the dimness hearing Peter's exasperated shouts from downstairs that his hammer was missing. He called upstairs asking my father if he'd picked it up. Leo was convinced that Peter had lost his mind since he'd seen him leave the hammer on the floor.

As Peter continued grumbling, Leo walked into our adjoined

bedrooms to check on the other builders and once inside my room he felt a compulsion to walk to the eyelid window and look across the garden. After scanning both sides, he looked down and noticed the wooden handle of something balancing on the window ledge below. It was a struggle to open the window as it was jammed by old paint and disrepair.

"Peter's hammer was balancing on the ledge. I couldn't move for a moment and just stared at it," he told me, still confounded.

The handle pointed outwards and someone would have had to first open the jammed window and then somehow reach down and across in order to balance the hammer precariously on the window ledge. Leo didn't dare retrieve the hammer and just walked downstairs to inform Peter where it was. What Peter made of this, I can only imagine.

Our father then walked out to his car and left. Unable to explain what he'd witnessed, he continued to dismiss stories of the paranormal.

6

FOOTBALL WITH
A PRIEST

It must have been an awkward telephone conversation for our mother to have with the local vicar of St Mary's Church at eleven o'clock that night. She'd thought of nothing else after the builders had given their account of why they had to abandon the cottage. According to Peter, it was more that the cottage had abandoned them. She'd waited as long as she could endure, wanting to speak to our father first, pacing up and down the bedroom cursing.

"You're always down the pub or working late or seeing a fucking colleague."

Alone and short-tempered with her nagging doubts, she gave up waiting and out of desperation looked up the number for the local vicarage. Conscious that it was now her duty, it seemed the most logical thing to do considering the strange circumstances she was confronting.

She also realised that Leo had kept her clueless about the occurrences in the cottage. With the facts in hand, she could piece together the details of my father's sporadic mumbling over the previous weeks. When he'd said, "I think the builders are going mad" or "What excuses will I hear today?", she was only being given the edited highlights about the goings-on. What troubled her most was not what she'd found out from the builders, but what she hadn't found out from her husband.

This further demonstrated our father's indifference. He was never there when she really needed him, whenever she needed solace or a voice of reason. With hindsight she felt foolish for ever considering him as being that kind of husband. Although indignant, she was curious why he hadn't told her the full story. What else was he keeping secret?

The repercussions seemed more disturbing as she thought about the wellbeing of us, her children. Then there was Sean's cupboard bedroom too. At eight feet square and built into the corner slope of the cottage roof, even Leo agreed it wasn't really suitable for a bedroom and an adult could barely stand inside. She considered it tantamount to neglect, putting a child into such a small windowless room, even temporarily. The cupboard bedroom was a further demonstration of Leo's reluctance to accept Sean and she wondered how much he even wanted his own children. She'd concluded long ago that Leo wasn't the paternal type. He was a war baby. When his own father had returned from the war to find his wife pandering to a new baby, their relationship began unsteadily and continued in the same way.

A warm, understanding voice answered the phone that night, soft and composed considering the late hour. Mum felt a welcome wave of relief.

"I'm not a believer," she began awkwardly. "What I mean is, I don't go to church."

Reverend Jones chuckled gently, telling her it was fine and inviting her to continue. Feeling calmer, Mum explained how she and her young family had only moved to the village a few weeks ago. She listed our names and ages. Jones must have considered her call as that of a new parishioner, lonely and disorientated with the transition between town and country. But as she finished telling him about us, her voice began to quiver. Sensing another agenda, he asked if she needed help in some way.

As Mum explained our current temporary living arrangements and the cottage renovations, she found herself unable to listen to her own babble and suddenly cut to the chase.

"I think there's something wrong with the cottage we're moving into. I think it might be haunted."

There was a pause as Reverend Jones contemplated this change of direction.

"Would you like me to come over in the morning for a chat?" he said.

"Thank you." Mum's voice trembled. "I hope you don't think I'm mad. Although… I've been having my doubts."

"Not at all." He surprised Mum again with his unfazed response. "I shouldn't really say this but, off the record, my wife is very spiritually gifted. I trust her perception implicitly when it comes to such matters."

It was arranged that he would collect the keys for the cottage in the morning, then he and his wife would make a visit to experience the atmosphere for themselves. Mum hoped that the Reverend and his wife would return and tell her everything was fine, she could live in Fir Tree Cottage without fear or worry. That way at least, she wouldn't have to approach the subject with her mother or her in-laws. How would she ever explain it to them?

When our father finally returned a short while after Mum had made the call, he looked at her in disbelief as she reproached him for not telling her the truth about the cottage. He seemed more exasperated by the news of the local clergy being engaged to help than the news of the builders abandoning the cottage. Confident he could coerce the builders back to finish the job with his natural gift of the gab, initially he didn't accept they'd left for good. But they never did return, despite his repeated attempts. Not only had they left their tools and belongings, they'd also bid farewell to a decent income.

After dropping us at our respective nursery and infant schools next morning, Mum returned to the bungalow to wait for Reverend Jones. She felt self-conscious as she replayed the conversation from the previous night, fearing she was losing touch as she stared at the cigarette trembling between her fingers.

When the Reverend arrived, he was wearing full regalia, his black cassock furling as he entered the gate as if about to give a sermon. It was a good thing that our father had already gone to work.

Jones greeted Mum with a warm smile. He was a large man and, by his slightly thinning fair hair, she estimated him to be in his early forties. She thought his rugged looks and bulky hands unusual for a man of the cloth, more suited to a farmer than a vicar. Once inside he said hello to Sean who gazed at him from his cot with curiosity.

"I'm going to pick up my wife shortly and we'll conduct an initial investigation," he said as he took the keys.

"Has your wife done anything like this before?" Mum asked, smiling timidly.

"The thing is," he answered quietly, "what I'm advocating here is frowned on by the Church. But if something is wrong with the cottage, my wife will be able to tell us. I trust her."

Mum says she found the idea of the Reverend using his wife as some paranormal barometer a bizarre concept. Yet she came to realise that Jones was gifted with the ability of nurturing his parishioners, with a formidable appetite for reaching out to everyone regardless of their spiritual persuasion. No, he didn't consider the paranormal his strong point. It wasn't that he didn't believe, but simply that his ministry decreed he left Spiritualism to others. Despite her convent education, Mum had no religious beliefs but she could tell that Reverend Jones was diligent, not a bigot, and an honest believer which she respected. She found herself envying his devout beliefs, the comfort of knowing there was, well, something other than this world.

"Remember that man talking about some weird satanic thing at the church, Marc?" Jason and I had been reliving some of the strangeness one afternoon.

A few years after moving to the area we'd overheard a story outside The Queen's Head one evening. Although our minds were susceptible to a fabricated tale, the parent of one of our friends later confirmed this one.

Hallowe'en trick-or-treating was catching on at the time and my brother and I recalled the novelty of knocking on the doors of strangers, hoping for the opportunity to inflict a trick. With my blacked-out face and novelty fangs, and Jason wearing a sheet over his head with holes cut out for eyes, we'd roamed the lanes with our few friends enjoying this new trend.

Early that particular October morning, the previous vicar had arrived at the churchyard, noticing an awful smell as he casually made his way towards the church entrance. The stench was alien to the normal sweet country air. In front of him, nailed to the wooden arch around the church door, was the bloody decapitated carcass of a goat. This was an occultist act of desecration rather than some macabre Hallowe'en prank. The shock sent him reeling, the peaceful quiet of the surrounding countryside in stark contrast to the gory scene before him. As the church was never locked at night, he was fearful of what he'd find inside, but relieved to find the church as untouched as he'd left it the previous evening.

It is common knowledge that among the gentry and bohemia in West Sussex there was a faction who enjoyed the solitude for other reasons. Indeed, paganists and occultists are still frequent visitors to Chanctonbury Ring, a prehistoric hill fort seven hundred feet above the coastline and some nine miles from our village. During the summer solstice, paganists hold secret ceremonies here as they've done for centuries. Similarly, during the Hallowe'en festivities, a more sinister faction hold their own ceremonies, making the most of this secluded area.

Reverend Jones and his wife unlocked the porch door to Fir Tree Cottage and entered the empty living room. Silently they assessed the atmosphere from their individual perspectives.

Now, I knew every inch of the cottage and I remember

its quirky foibles. The vicar's wife would have struggled to remain objective of what she perceived that morning when she first entered. Sunlight passing through the uneven leaded glass triangles casts strange, diffracted shadows across the walls giving the illusion of movement within the emptiness. Shards of illuminated dust contributed further to this uncanny illusion. Whistling breezes would send flutters of soot down the chimney into the hearth. Draughts slipped through the gaps around the windows and creaking doors. It was easy to evoke something from your imagination within the apparent beauty of Fir Tree Cottage.

The cold coupled with the faint scent of damp was to be expected, as was the sense of abandonment. The cottage was empty now. As the vicar's wife took in the wraps of tools on the dusty floorboards, jackets hooked on the mantle above the fireplace and the shoes arranged inside the porch door, she could see that beyond the emptiness was a testimony to fear of happenings still unexplained.

Reverend Jones went to walk through the open doors to the stairwell, his bulk filling the gloomy aperture, but his wife immediately told him not to go any further. She looked inside the door to the left of the fireplace and down onto the empty room below. It was clean now, the smell of fresh paint permeating the space. Looking through the front window, she noticed the barren earth covering the area where the pond had once been. The place seemed clean but something still lingered somewhere and she sensed it.

She told her husband she didn't want to go upstairs. She wanted to leave the cottage straight away and she was already certain of one thing. For his part, Reverend Jones would give his backing to whatever she decided. He didn't question what she felt for he could also sense, beyond the drabness, some kind of peculiarity.

As they pulled up outside, my mother came to the door anxiously. She was surprised by how little time they'd spent at the cottage. Was it a good sign? She hadn't met the vicar's wife and didn't know how to read her sheepish expression. Was she trembling?

"Was everything okay?" Mum asked apprehensively.

The vicar suggested they sit in the lounge to discuss things. It was evident they had both made a decision. Mum told me she remembers how impatient she was; the burning question was whether we could all move into our forever home. The initial signs didn't look good. Reverend Jones was holding his wife's hand gently as she looked at my mother with compassion.

"I sensed something small and evil at the cottage," she then said clearly. "You shouldn't go and live there with the children yet."

There was a long pause while Mum took in this shocking statement.

"What am I going to do?" she asked. The question she'd harboured ever since the builders left emerged as an anguished plea and again she questioned her own sanity.

"There's someone I need to talk to within the Church," said the Reverend. "He's very well regarded in these matters."

"Who's that?" Mum asked, trembling with emotion.

"Dom Robert Petitpierre."

As we talked this over, Jason sat slumped in his chair staring at the carpet, the abstract pattern of stains as unfathomable as his mind.

"Yeah," he nodded slowly. "I remember Dom Robert clearly. He was a really nice bloke wasn't he?"

"It amazes me what you still remember, Jace," I said, taking out my laptop. I began reading out the draft of this chapter, to see what else my brother would recover from his past.

Jason twisted my arm behind my back and pushed me against the wall of the lean-to. At four years-old he was still a lot smaller than me, but when playing Batman he was endowed with special powers. That was the rule and we stuck to it religiously despite our size difference.

Every fight scene re-enacted was performed in slow motion with each punch, kick or chop landing like a feather on a pillow. Each KAPOW Jason made as he placed a punch tenderly on the point of my chin was followed by my theatrical ARRGH. A kick landed with a POW was followed by my groaning UGGH as I crumpled to the ground dramatically, clutching my solar plexus. The battles would be spontaneous and could last for hours although sometimes our skirmishes were limited to the brief period between swapping over who played in goal.

"Let's play football again," I said. I picked myself up from the damp grass and moved Jason's tatty parka jacket nearer to the other goalpost, my grey check tank top, which I hated. I'd do this sneaky trick to make the goalmouth smaller and give me an advantage whenever Jason's back was turned as he dribbled the football away down the garden. Our sorry-looking pitch on the lawn was still mostly earth where the old pond used to be.

Our youthful exuberance afforded us natural immunity from the cold when we played outside during winter. It was just as well this particular day as we were under strict instructions to remain outside the cottage. Our parents had informed us that some special people were coming to visit, people who were going to help Mum get the cottage ready for us to live in. Although curious, we didn't complain. Our parents had effectively scored an own goal by imploring us to keep out; the garden was what we liked best about the cottage. Staying indoors made us feel sad and edgy.

In goal I performed my usual routine. I adjusted my yellow football socks, the only piece of football kit I owned, an homage to my football hero, Pelé. Jason waited patiently, adjusting his glasses and squinting, his tongue protruding slightly. Then with a single bounce I kicked the ball clumsily between the top of my foot and my shin, propelling it high into the air towards the maze of barren rhododendrons in the lower half of the garden. The ball crashed through the branches like a small bomb. We always agreed, whenever we discussed these games in later life, that I was really bad at football.

"That was rubbish," Jason exclaimed, running towards the dense thicket. After several minutes of frantic rustling, my brother emerged victorious with the ball but then came to an abrupt halt, his focus on a car we didn't recognise entering the driveway.

We watched the beige Austin crunch its way up the driveway and coast past us. There were two men inside, both looking formal and slightly scary as we stared at them through the car windows. From their aura of formality we knew these must be the special people our parents had referred to, the ones who were going to help Mum with the cottage.

The car stopped just short of the patio. The older man climbed from the passenger side first before the younger man exited. We recognised from their clothes that they were holy men, priests of some description. Our curiosity heightened as we observed our mother and father waiting awkwardly in front of the cottage.

The younger man smiled at us before approaching my parents. Our eyes were fixated on the older man who hadn't acknowledged us yet, as he looked beyond the patio and silently surveyed the cottage. We walked towards him, wondering if we were in some way invisible, Jason still clutching the ball under his arm.

This man was an oddity in his black dress and presented an almost sinister figure, especially when he turned back to the car and reached inside to retrieve a few random items: an old book and a silver receptacle, along with some pieces of folded cloth. As he turned and smiled at my brother, we realised we were not invisible to him after all, and his withered, characterful face was full of charisma. He was a slight man of medium height, well groomed, with grey swept-back hair.

"Hello chaps," he greeted us warmly before crossing the lawn where he stood and perused the grave of the old pond. Turning back to us, he asked, "What are your names then, my good fellows?"

Placing a hand on my brother's head he looked at him patiently as my brother said, "I'm Jason."

"And I'm Marc," I said confidently, taking a failed swipe towards the ball my brother clutched under his arm. The ball bounced softly, landing at the feet of the priest. "Who are you?" I asked.

"My name is Dom Robert Petitpierre." He sounded out each syllable of his surname slowly, before prodding the ball with the point of his toe. A grin stretched across Jason's face. "Right then! Who fancies a game of footy?"

We looked at the priest with excitement and confusion; he was a riddle we were unable to comprehend. The sight of this ancient man wearing a flowing black dress and white collar seemed as absurd to us as it was delightful. Jason began giggling as the priest dribbled the ball towards us. "Come on," he said. "Who's going to take the ball from me?"

I cannot remember any other moment when I have seen my brother so animated as when the priest turned his back and headed towards our parka and tank top goalposts. Jason rushed at Petitpierre as he dribbled the ball across the lumpy earth. I watched Jason giggle, hacking purposeful feints at the ball in an effort to regain possession. I've no recollection of my brother ever playing football with that same vigour, his concentration total, his happiness tangible. Finally, Jason resorted to pulling the flowing tails of the priest's frock in an effort to curtail him. My brother's oafish efforts were in vain though. The priest tapped the ball into a low arch and it slapped against the whitewashed wall of the garage lean-to like a heavy wet fish.

"Goooooaal!" He grinned, playfully pumping his arms in the air as he performed his victory parade. We both jumped around him laughing, pulling at his dress, daring ourselves to rough play with this holy stranger.

Dom Robert Petitpierre was one of the warmest and friendliest adults we'd ever encountered. It struck us as odd that a man so old could possess more fun and energy than our father, a considerably younger man who never interacted with us much.

"Why have you come to our new house?" Jason asked, with that screwed-up expression of confusion on his face he always had when asking questions.

"I've come with my friend, Reverend Jones, to bless your house," he said and cupped our faces gently with his sinewy hands. This kind familiarity was alien to us.

"Is that a good thing?" I enquired seriously.

"Yes, it's a good thing!" Dom Robert replied. "Now, why don't you two go and practise your football while we pop inside and talk to your mother and father. We'll be out in a short while."

We nodded obediently and watched the two cloaked figures mount the steps to the patio and disappear inside the cottage.

7

THE REVEREND AND
THE IRREVERENT

Years later, I spent several days talking to my mother about the events of that day and, along with a rare copy of Petitpierre's autobiography, I stitched together the following account.

Reverend Jones led Dom Robert into the lounge where my parents were waiting pensively.

"Would you like some tea?" Mum asked, unsure how to conduct herself.

"Thank you, yes. It's pretty darn cold in here." Dom Robert blew into his hands. "You must be Carol? And you must be Leo?" He smiled at my mother before shaking my father's hand. My mother felt apprehensive and clutched her Silk Cut as she went to make the drinks. My father, in stark contrast, appeared indifferent. He was impeccably dressed as ever and clearly preoccupied with other agendas that should have been filling his day.

Having warmed up with some tea and small talk, Dom Robert placed an ancient book on the mantelpiece. My mother remembers that at this point his face seemed strangely familiar to her, enhancing the sense of reassurance and trust she felt about this curious stranger.

"I know this may all seem rather mediaeval, a stuffy monk coming to your house in the middle of the day to conduct some sort of strange ritual," Dom Robert began. "I'm not going

71

to do anything weird or fabulous and exciting. I just want to walk around the grounds initially, to get a feel of what's taking place here." He glanced across at Reverend Jones. "Now, is the builder fellow coming today, Reverend? Peter, I think you said his name was?"

The Reverend shook his head, looking towards my father for confirmation.

"Basically he's refused point blank to have anything more to do with the cottage, the work or, indeed, me," Leo declared rolling his eyes, not quite believing his own summary of the current events. Our father was resolute that under no circumstances would he ever adopt any paranormal beliefs, unlike the collection of overzealous loons surrounding him. He'd made this point particularly clear to my mother. Dom Robert remained unmoved by the unspoken challenge.

"Now, Carol," he said, "I know the Reverend has briefly told you my itinerary but I wanted to make sure you're okay for me to proceed and walk around the grounds to perform my initial blessing?"

"Is it all right for the boys to remain outside?" Mum asked anxiously, realising she hadn't understood the itinerary at all.

"This initial blessing should be natural and low key, so please let them continue playing outside. That's precisely what we need." He reached inside his cassock and retrieved various items before placing a stole around his neck. Retrieving a glass flask of holy water, he placed it beside his book on the mantelpiece.

As my mother watched these ceremonial preparations, the energy of the room seemed to gain potency, making her feel more apprehensive. She couldn't help asking one of the many questions tumbling around her mind.

"Reverend Jones tells me you're experienced with these things?" Not quite knowing herself what 'these things' actually were, she continued, "Sorry if it's a strange question, but how did you become involved with ghosts and stuff?"

"It's not a strange question at all, Carol. A lot of people think of exorcisms, spiritual existence, ghosts and the like with either ridicule or hysteria. There's been little scientific study of the subject until recent times. I was part of a team of theologians and clergy convened to write a study into this area. The idea was to try and de-demonise the ritual and help to explain what the spiritual realm means to us as Christians."

Mum nodded, pretending she understood as my father turned away with a look of ill-concealed disdain. Before he could say something contemptuous, Dom Robert continued expounding his position.

"For me, the ritual of exorcism is a way of demonstrating the enduring power of the Holy Spirit in giving us the power to overcome evil in the world. In layman's terms, it's a guide to spiritual warfare."

Another superior smile spread across our father's face as he glanced around the room, observing Reverend Jones and his own wife, musing to himself, 'They surely don't believe this bollocks do they?' He rolled his eyes and turned to look outside, watching us zigzagging around the garden in pursuit of the ball.

"Of course," Dom Robert continued, observing Leo knowingly, "I've been around on this Earth a while now. I'm a servant of God, but I know that to many people, regrettably, this notion of spiritual warfare is simply nonsense. The world is increasingly fixated on material possessions, media and tabloids. Now the notion of being created by a God wanting to bring us in from darkness seems like ancient superstition. Mankind has lost sight of the spiritual realm."

He picked up the Bible from the mantelpiece and opened it. Cupping it carefully in his hands, he read out a short paragraph.

"Romans, Chapter One, verse twenty-two. 'Professing themselves to be wise, they became fools.'" Looking across the room, he sighed. "I think that quotation perfectly describes the way mankind has blinded itself with the belief that science can explain everything." Closing the Bible, he tucked it away within his cassock. "And coming from a former scientist, that really is some statement," he chuckled. "I actually studied to be a chemist initially, not a theologian. I studied at Merton College, Oxford. That was when I experienced my first exorcism, within the college, performed by a friend who was an undergraduate Anglican priest."

"What happened?" Mum asked, eyes wide with intrigue.

A man dressed in Tudor costume had appeared in the dormitories, witnessed by several fellow students and causing considerable agitation within the faculty. Dom Robert described the appearances, rather peculiarly, as, "A typical intelligent, paranormal haunting... a ghost proper."

"How do you mean, 'intelligent'?" Mum asked, trying to conceal her initial amusement.

"What many people do not understand is that sometimes, when one sees a physical form or what may be called a ghost, it is in fact just a residue – like a scene from the past inexplicably replayed... a sort of movie. If this sounds far-fetched, consider the technology we have nowadays. We have infrared apparatus that can detect the imprint of an aircraft hours after it has taken off. In a way, it's the same principle.

"This sort of random entity never displays any awareness of their present-day observers whatsoever, hence the term unintelligent. It's simply a memory immortalised in time. Whereas in the case I've mentioned the spectre was human-like and displayed a certain level of personality and emotion, such as unhappiness. And it was obviously responding to changes around it."

"But it's not actual intelligence, is it?" Mum giggled nervously, spilling the last of her tea onto the floorboards and hoping Dom Robert didn't think she was mocking him. He merely raised his eyebrows.

"Sometimes entities have been known to write messages, you know. Often with typical paranormal, intelligent hauntings, the phenomena are brought about by changes to the inside of a building or the grounds. This suggests these beings may have once lived in the place before becoming lost in the afterlife in some way. By intelligent, I mean that they are attempting to respond to these changes. They're aware of this dimension as well as their own. Generally, they convey dissatisfaction and sadness."

"So can they make noises and move things around? That can terrify people, like our builders."

"Certainly, my dear. In a place haunted by an intelligent entity, phenomenon are not purely visual. Some people are more attuned to visual occurrences, others more attuned to sounds, even disembodied voices."

"So what happened during the first ritual you experienced?" Mum asked, feeling a chill run through her.

Dom Robert described how he'd assisted his friend along with another student, performing the ritual through the window of his friend's room overlooking the quadrangle of the college. The undergraduate priest read the ritual to command the spirit to depart in the name of Christ.

"I really didn't believe in what I was doing at the time, believe it or not. I wanted to be involved out of curiosity more than anything else. But then, without warning, everything in the room began to shake and rattle. It was most alarming. My friend's washstand seemed as though it would fall off the wall." Although unemotional, Dom Robert was clearly still shocked about what happened that day.

"I came away knowing there really was no other explanation. After we'd completed the ceremony, I'm pleased to say there were no further hauntings. So after my Chemistry degree I found myself studying Theology at St Paul's Missionary College in Lincolnshire. Quite a transformation, I'm sure you'll agree."

My mother realised he was giving an honest account, at the same time acknowledging that her own perception of reality now had blurred edges.

"Have you actually ever seen a ghost?" she asked.

"Only one, in a church near City Road in London. But it's generally not what I see that gives me my conclusions about a particular case, Carol, it's what I sense as I survey a place. Information I receive through the unconscious mind."

Mum looked again at our father to see if he was taking in any of this information and watched him staring unresponsively into the garden again.

"They're lovely boys," commented Dom Robert, following his gaze. "Obviously very curious about all this, so I'll try and make the initial blessing very quick and simple. Please remain in the lounge while we walk around the grounds. We should only be ten minutes or so."

He gave Reverend Jones a knowing nod. Then he took the small glass flask from the mantelpiece, removed the pewter top and walked towards the porch, dispensing a sprinkle of water onto the floorboards before stepping outside onto the patio. Reading from the Mozarabic Rite, Dom Robert spoke in a calm, commanding tone.

"God, the Son of God, who by death destroyed death, and overcame him who had the power over death, beat down Satan quickly. Amen."

The two men descended the steps of the patio and walked across the driveway towards the lawn. Seeing the cloaked figures approaching and presuming another game was about to ensue, we disappeared around the back of the lean-to and hid among the dead ferns and branches. From our hideout, we watched silently as they walked slowly down to the furthest corner of the garden, down the slope where the rope swing hung. The smaller man, who'd played football with us, walked a few feet in front of the taller holy man. It was like viewing a movie. The contrast between the man who'd previously played football and the serious man now muttering to himself, captivated our attention as he waved his hand at various areas of the garden.

Inside the cottage our parents looked out of the window and watched them at work, my mother half-expecting to see an apparition herself, my father wanting desperately for the two apparitions he could see to piss off and go home. Leo looked at his watch. It was only eleven-thirty.

"What time have we got to endure this again this evening?" he asked crossly.

"Seven o'clock," Mum snapped.

Whereas I remember a dusty haze in the garden that morning, a light mist that inhibited my vision, Jason shared a different perspective with me.

"I remember this feeling in the garden like a vacuum, which came down like a cloud and made everything silent. Even the birds stopped singing." He was convinced of this, another of his indelible memories he couldn't obliterate no matter how hard he tried. As the two men passed the garage lean-to and moved into the back garden, we continued to watch them, certain they weren't aware of us.

"O God, the Author of blessing and Fount of salvation, we earnestly pray and beseech You to pour the manifold dew of Your grace and the abundance of Your blessing upon this place. Amen," Dom Robert pronounced assertively.

We listened, wondering what the words meant. The taller man was watching him vigilantly at all times and occasionally spoke, although the shorter man seemed oddly oblivious of his conversation.

Mum stood in the centre in the lounge as the two men came back inside the cottage, uncertain of her role. While they had been outside doing whatever it was they did, she'd been in a quandary, wondering whether she should pray reverently. And now, should she continue playing the concerned hostess? Her unease was made harder by her husband's petulant tutting and disbelieving glances at his wristwatch.

"It was a bit sticky out there while I performed the blessing," observed Dom Robert. Mum says she has often contemplated this remark since; what did he mean by 'sticky'? "Do you know you have gooseberry bushes in the right-hand corner of the garden?" he added jovially. Both my parents shook their heads, perplexed.

"I'm certain that whatever's happening started outside and

was brought into this cottage inadvertently by the builder fellow, Peter." Dom Robert looked out of the window and muttered, "It's a shame he couldn't be here, it would have been of great help. I think our man Peter is a chaotic psychic. I mean, he has no way of controlling his abilities and most probably is unable to comprehend them at all."

At this, in a rare moment of solidarity, my parents agreed they had no idea what Dom Robert was talking about. He then turned from the window and addressed them directly. As though reading the findings of a property survey, he matter-of-factly presented his case regarding what he believed was at work, what he thought was responsible for driving the builders from the cottage in terror.

"Well, I believe the figure that was seen in the garden and indeed inside these walls was a genuine ghost, perhaps a tramp who had once used the bridlepath. It's likely he resented the changes being made to the cottage and grounds."

This statement hit my parents squarely on the jaw. For Mum, it was as if she'd been told that fairies really do exist and now found herself inexplicably believing in them. For our indignant father, it was the opposite. To have a man, undoubtedly a learned and holy man, tell him so blatantly that a ghost was roaming around his property wasn't only laughable, it was an insult to his own substantial intelligence. He would have imagined that he would only have to endure a ridiculous bout of rapturous hymns and prayers before all these zealots would just fuck off and leave him to get on with the business of somehow completing his dream renovation. But now there was a prognosis for the perceived problem, one apparently needing a cure, and he found himself starting to despair.

"I believe the foreman, Peter, caused a lot of the poltergeist disturbances himself, inadvertently of course," Dom Robert continued, ignoring the incredulous looks from my father. "This was pure chaotic psychic energy. Children are very often the culprits actually, not adults.

"Poltergeist activity can be unsettling but I've never

experienced a case where anyone has been actually harmed. Alarmed, yes, but never harmed." He turned to my mother with a look of reassurance. "I believe a lot of what disturbed the builders here was directly attributed to Peter. However, some of the happenings were undoubtedly the result of the ghost. For example, our spirit here, I'm inclined to believe, was probably responsible for the fire being extinguished."

My mother began to comprehend now that there seemed to be two paranormal incidences at work. One of them, she hoped naïvely, would not make a reappearance now that Peter had fled.

"So why do we have to have a second ceremony?" she asked.

"I purely tested the water out there." Dom Robert motioned to the garden with his hand. "Exorcism can only be employed against evil coming into the world from outside, so to speak. Non-human spirits, not manifestations that are a direct result of human psychic energy." He spoke slowly, observing our parents to see if his explanation was being understood. "Generally, poltergeist activity cannot be cured by sacraments of any kind. However, if the disturbance is generated by a departed and disruptive spirit, often Holy Communion or Requiem Mass can release the soul. There is also the danger of infiltration by evil – little devils if you like – so I like to be thorough and conduct a full service of exorcism if I'm unsure."

The priest touched my mother's hand in an act of reassurance. If he was bothered about my father's obvious scepticism, he didn't react. He had his work to complete regardless. Mum's mind whirled over 'non-human spirit' and 'little devils' apprehensively, struggling to accept that she was starting to believe.

The interior of the cottage was to be cleansed that evening. By seven o'clock, Dom Robert Petitpierre had erected a small makeshift altar in the middle of the kitchen, a white cloth draped over a small table. On this he'd placed his silk stole, his flask of holy water and an old Bible along with another book of sacraments.

Standing silently alongside my father and Reverend Jones, still in full regalia, Mum imagined the likelihood of the inexplicable making an actual appearance. The fantasy, however startling, also had a certain appeal: she wanted this… whatever it was… to reveal itself. That would teach him. She imagined Leo's belligerence turning to terror if the ghost of Fir Tree Cottage shouted and screamed in the way Peter had described. How quickly would he flee the house?

"Thank you for your hospitality and cooperation." Dom Robert smiled at his small congregation. "Before I start cleaning up the rest of the muck here I would like to start with the Lord's Prayer." He bowed his head along with the vicar and they both recited it forcefully with reverence. Mum could only remember saying the 'Our Father' bit before uttering 'Amen' at the end, while Leo looked down at his feet for the duration and admired his boots.

Reverend Jones was to remain in the kitchen with my parents while Dom Robert went around the cottage and visited each room. He gathered up the holy water and his books, walked to the door of the kitchen and before leaving turned to read from the Mozarabic Rite.

"O God, the Author of blessing and Fount of salvation, we earnestly pray and beseech You to pour the manifold dew of Your grace and the abundance of Your blessing upon this place. Amen." As he sprinkled the floor with some of the water, Mum braced herself, believing that if anything was going to happen it could be now.

He walked across to the doors of the stairway and, as he opened them, the creak pierced the stillness of the evening. He sprinkled his water again.

"May You grant it prosperity and drive out adversity. Amen." As he passed through the doors, his words dulled as he made his way up the stairs. "May You drive out Satan, the author of evil. Amen."

When he reached the foot of the landing, his words became muffled beyond recognition as the protesting floorboards creaked in the direction of the furthest bedroom. Meanwhile, in the kitchen Reverend Jones looked to be in prayer, his head bowed. My mother made a conscious effort not to look at her husband.

Within a few minutes, the monk's footsteps were above them as he now stood in the bathroom. Mum remembered Peter's haunted face as he'd told her of the figure leering at him through the mirror there. She shuddered, wondering what, if anything, Dom Robert was now confronting. Listening carefully, she could hear only his murmurings above. She waited in expectation of a change of pitch, for the mumblings to perhaps change from a steady drone to a wail, a frightened scream, and for pandemonium to erupt. But she only heard the steady rhythmic sound of his voice and the floorboards' frequent creaks as he shuffled around the tiny bathroom. He stayed there for quite some time before his footsteps gained pace, making their way towards the adjoined bedrooms of her children.

Mum thought about her children, hoping that her mother-in-law was coping with my exuberance and Jason's quiet reservation. Was Sean asleep yet? She was glad we were safely out of the way, a ten-minute drive away. All she wanted was for the cottage to be deemed a safe place to bring her family to live.

It was almost twenty minutes before she finally heard Dom Robert's footsteps descend the stairs, his words once again coming into range as he emerged through the stair doors and into the lounge.

"By the multitude of Your mercies, may peace abound for those who dwell in this place. Amen." He walked around the corner towards the furthest corner of the room. "Send, O Lord, to this dwelling Your good and holy angel. Amen."

His voice sounded, says my mother, as though he was forcibly rousing himself, trying to muster his courage. She watched him leave the room and descend the short stairs to the adjoined garage, the last room of the house where again his words became muffled. Sensing the ceremony was coming to an end, Mum felt her breathing become less shallow and she allowed herself to relax a little. Whatever she thought, or perhaps hoped, might happen had not materialised. Outside the evening was still.

Dom Robert stumbled through the doors of the adjoined garage and back into the lounge, sprinkling the last of his holy water. The others all recognised his look of depletion as he moved slowly towards the kitchen, a shadow of his former vigorous self. Clearly in distress, he wiped his brow before placing his tools on the altar and looking up at his congregation, unable to smile.

"It was putting up some resistance. It was quite a struggle actually." He looked surprised as well as tired, and as Reverend Jones went to help with dismantling the altar, he stumbled again. The Reverend placed his arm under Dom Robert's forearm to support him as his legs wilted.

"If you wouldn't mind," he said to our parents, "we'd like you to come back to the vicarage for some refreshments." He looked at them hopefully and my father got the message.

"I remember Mum telling someone," Jason told me, animated as though the event had happened yesterday not decades before, "that Leo had to help Dom Robert to his car. Apparently he was quite shocked." My brother smiled with a look of curious satisfaction.

At the vicarage later, my parents found Reverend Jones and Dom Robert drinking tea in the living room. The vicar's wife greeted them. My mother was slightly amused by the thought of finally having tea at a vicarage, whilst our father was less enthralled. However, since helping the monk out of the cottage, his petulance had subsided and he more readily accepted these final formalities. Dom Robert appeared to have recovered his strength.

"The cause of so many of the disturbances I encounter these days," he commented, as though to reassure our parents, "are human in their origin. So often it's the case that the person most disturbed by a phenomenon is the person who caused it. When people dabble in dangerous stuff they don't understand, such as Ouija boards, is where it all goes wrong for them and things get messy."

He was referring to Peter of course, and the whistles and strange sounds he'd experienced, the builders' voices being mimicked. But could an otherwise ordinary man really exude the energy to manufacture all of the paranormal behaviour the men collectively experienced? Mum felt the whirl of another million questions she wanted to ask him, but could only think of the obvious one.

"Everything should be fine now," the monk replied. "I've cleared up all the muck." He smiled and lifted his cup to his lips.

An hour later, as they drove back to the bungalow, Mum considered the day's events and remembers thinking that the monk's eccentric terminology seemed a little superficial and not the wholehearted reassurance she had first sought. But then, how could anyone really profess fully to comprehend that which is beyond comprehension?

Quite what 'muck' had been 'cleared up' she could only imagine. And what had been left behind would later became an unending debate.

A few years later, Dom Robert Petitpierre's own account of his experience at Fir Tree Cottage was featured in several tabloid newspapers. He was even interviewed by the late John Peel, and eventually became something of a minor celebrity in his own unassuming way.

8

ONE FINAL BATTLE

It was a Saturday morning in January when Mum drove us to begin our new life at the cottage. Our father was going to follow on later, he'd informed her, although I have no memory of him arriving that day. The delights of the garden aside, we were nervous as my mother crunched the car carefully up the driveway. We set eyes on the cottage again knowing, no matter what, this was where we would be living forever as we'd been told on far too many occasions.

Our first impressions left an indelible feeling in us both, though we each have different recollections of why. Mine was more a sense of uncertainty, something ominous that mostly made me feel unsettled. But I guess all children might well experience the same sort of thing especially when moving into a new home. This unsettled sensation was often present during all the years we lived there. Jason's recollections, however, still haunt him to this day.

As a precaution for the day, Mum had equipped us with a selection of favourite toys, hoping they'd sooth any anxiety and entertain us sufficiently while she began the ominous task of single-handedly transforming the cottage into something resembling a home.

We stood outside on the patio full of trepidation as Mum,

clutching Sean in one arm, pushed open the porch and front doors, mustering every ounce of enthusiasm she could for this new adventure we were embarking upon. Knowing the emptiness waiting inside, she hoped that we'd only see a brighter hope for our future rather than the present empty relic. You had to hand it to her. She had unbending fortitude, which I have often mistaken since for plain stubbornness.

Jason and I looked around at the undressed lounge and considered the bare floorboards dejectedly. There were only two simple wooden chairs furnishing the room, which we didn't recognise as anything we'd owned previously. The windows had no curtains and the whole interior exuded emptiness and abandonment as we stared at the cold ash mound in the fireplace. Our mother managed to contain her own deep disappointment and maintained her enthusiastic charade for our benefit.

Inside, however, she nurtured further resentment towards our father for not being present to offer solidarity in carrying off this illusion of hope for her kids. She recalls the additional anxiety heaped upon her of whether the removals van would arrive at all, let alone in time for her to salvage the day for us.

We all remember the removals man with fondness. Bill had already become a family friend we considered a kindly uncle. His affable weathered face we'd often find grinning at us when we shinned the barrel delivery hatch of The Queen's Head and pressed our faces to the window to plead for a Coke. Bill was a lovely man. Considered a permanent fixture of the pub, he generally contemplated the world through the bottom of a pint glass. Now all our personal belongings were stored in the back of his truck with the slurred promise from the previous night that he'd turn up at the agreed time of 'some point in the morning'.

Inside the lounge, we stood trying to comprehend how the inside of the cottage managed to be as cold as the outside. That wasn't the way we understood a home should work. But we knew this was it, there was no turning back and we'd have to make the most of it. The idea of this being a forever home was a daunting prospect especially against the backdrop of our parents' volatility.

Our mother was desperate to keep us busy with chores that first day, like letting us furnish our bedrooms, badly in need of the homely touches of toys, books, games and bedclothes. The simple things that turn a space into a place. Getting us to settle in bed on that first night was going to be a monumental struggle that she dreaded.

Eventually, the house was made homely, we went to school and tried settling into a normal life. The garden became our best friend amidst the growing anguish between our parents.

"I didn't really know what normal was then, I guess," Jason reflected about this time. "Kids adapt, don't they? Even to things they maybe shouldn't have to." With two gulps, Jason drank his coffee.

One spring day, I had stood on the patio outside the kitchen window frozen by indecision. My brother recounted his own memory of this defining moment.

"I ran downstairs from my room when I heard Mum crying in pain." Even as Jason gave his account of that day he still showed the fearful hurt of a sensitive child, his fist gripped tightly as though still clutching his Action Man. "I looked towards the kitchen where I heard grunting and swearing going on and saw Mum being pulled across the kitchen by her hair before being shook like a rag doll. I'll never forget her crying out, pleading for me to go and get the neighbour, Mr Stevens."

We had a retired neighbour who'd occasionally pop his head over the fence and have a friendly conversation with us. Mum often talked to this older man, a reliable father figure with a voice of reason. To us, he was a friendly stranger but to our mother at this moment he was the only adult she knew who could possibly be strong enough to end the fiasco and spare her children from the hatred filling our home. Jason was clearly in shock, as he appeared from the porch onto the patio, tears already brimming.

"Mum needs help. She said to get Mr Stevens." Clutching two Action Men close to his chest, his face was a veil of fear and confusion.

"Wait over there, Jace." I pointed to the rope swing.

"Will it be alright?" He asked tearfully. I nodded uncertainly as another tirade erupted behind us.

"You fucking bitch."

Jason ran like a whippet across the lawn to the other end of the garden, fingers in his ears, unable to listen to the anger between our parents any longer. Upstairs in his cupboard bedroom, Sean played alone, also hoping the erupting argument would end. For myself, I hadn't a clue what the words I heard through the window actually meant. As our parents wailed furiously around the kitchen table, the dog locked in their bedroom for safekeeping barked at them with a rival rage.

"I know you've been sleeping with her so don't fucking lie to me." Our mother's guttural words were so violent it was as though she was spitting out chunks of our father's flesh. I was scared of her when she was like this, angry and unpredictable, a dangerous creature. "She's eighteen, no more than a child, but that wouldn't stop you, would it?"

Our father tried protesting his innocence, saying he was simply fond of the girl in question, the village Carnival Queen and daughter of a local antique dealer. This didn't wash. Mum had heard too many rumours about them, some she'd ignored and others she simply couldn't.

From my viewpoint on the patio, Mum seemed to be turning the tables and gaining the upper hand in this latest conflict. With dreadful curiosity I stood paralysed, trying to distinguish exactly who was doing what to whom behind the leaded panes. It was highly probable their fighting would extend beyond the morning and last way into the evening. Should I do as Jason said and go and get the neighbour?

At the other end of the garden, Jason descended the slope on the rope swing, jumping high and long, disappearing from view behind the dense rhododendrons. He was in his happier place, I believed, away from the oppression inside and I felt relieved he was out of earshot. I'd already done enough damage myself that Christmas. During a moment of pompous self-belief I'd decided that Jason, at six, needed to confront the painful truth about Santa. I'd grown sick of the endless rhetoric about Father Christmas coming soon and the ensuing threat it entailed if we didn't clean our rooms and behave well.

My legs turned to jelly as Mum gave a piercing scream. From their silhouetted shapes I could make out my mother being shaken by her hair. Our father made full use of his new advantage. Following another stifled squeal, he growled at her triumphantly and forced me into an unenviable quandary. I knew something drastic and immediate needed to be done. Meanwhile, inside the kitchen Mum began sobbing with pain before once again rallying to her own defence. I admired her fighting spirit.

Jason now stood motionless at the top of the slope looking as though he might run and fetch the neighbour after all. I felt helpless about how to spare him from this ugly turmoil between our parents.

"You fucking bastard," she exclaimed with a distorted growl, as though her face was being pushed against a hard surface, or perhaps being pinched. Should I wait out the fracas on the end of the rope swing with Jason or charge into the kitchen like an eight year-old superhero to save Mum? The decision was made unexpectedly by something smashing through the kitchen window. The chipped ashtray sent a shower of shards tinkling around my feet like tiny meteorites.

My mind went blank as adrenalin took control. I rushed through the porch knowing the time to intervene had come, although not quite sure what my action should be. Inside, Mum was a figure of calmness. She was an enigma, often emotional and pushed to despair by her calamitous marriage, yet sometimes she was clinically calm. Her pretence prevented me from venturing directly into the war zone. And it was evident she had hatched a plan.

"Get Jason and wait in the car," she instructed me with the serenity of a mother about to tell a bedtime story. There were times when we knew not to dare question her orders and just obey. This was one such time.

Obediently I cupped my hands to my mouth and shouted across the garden to Jason. My brother rushed from behind the rhododendrons, timid and pale, twigs sticking out of his jumper, a fully equipped Action Man gripped in his hands. He'd tried not to listen to the hatred but the side effects were already showing. He followed me to the car, tearful and too terrified to ask questions, and stared at me in the rear view mirror, stroking the bristled hair on the head of his toy.

Our mother emerged, obliterating the calm as she screamed more unintelligible words at our father hiding inside the cottage. She picked up something from the front garden before reappearing above the patio wall and dashing towards us. Clutching Sean against her chest, she placed him in the back seat alongside Jason before closing the car door.

"Hold onto this for me please," she asked calmly, pulling my door open and placing something heavy wrapped in a towel on my lap. Then she ran round and threw herself into the driver's seat, started the engine and crunched the Mini into gear.

"Where are we going, Mum?" Jason's frightened voice bleated from the back seat like a spring lamb. Looking down at the collection of rocks in the towel I was holding, I had a more pressing question.

"What are these for, Mum?" I asked in total confusion.

She had the same expression of unconditional focus as Jason's scarred Action Man as she yanked on the handbrake at the foot of the drive. Then, with the engine still running, she hopped from the car like a ballerina, opened my door and gathered the towel containing the rocks.

"I won't be long," she said as she marched purposefully across the lawn towards the cottage.

The first rock she launched at the kitchen window hit its target with the precision of an Exocet missile. Our mouths gaped and I watched Jason's terror in the mirror. Jason was often unnerved inside the cottage, but now outside his anxiety had spiralled into overload, tears trickling down his cheeks as he tried to shield himself behind his Action Man.

Mum shifted across the patio following her target on the other side of the windows and fired another rock. The piercing sound of smashing glass filled the lane. We shrank fearfully into our seats. With breathtaking dexterity she paced across the patio firing the remaining three rocks in quick succession, each hitting the windows dead centre with a popping smash.

Jason was frozen in horror. We'd never seen our mother do anything with such athleticism or loathing.

"When Mum put those rocks through the window, I knew Dad would soon be going forever," Jason said forlornly, still picturing that chaotic day with grief years later. "I wanted to not be there anymore. I wanted everything to be peaceful without the hatred and shouting. If I'd have known about the gear then, I'd probably have started earlier."

Mum dropped the towel and sprinted back to the car wide-eyed, her composure gone. Launching herself inside, she threw down the handbrake and reversed into the lane like a rally driver. From the porch we caught a brief glimpse of our father watching us depart, hands thrashing the air with exaggerated anger.

Mum's resolve expired completely as she exited the lane outside our cottage. She hadn't a clue where to head, navigating through a curtain of tears she was desperate to deny. Jason watched with tearful dread, clutching her arm through the seat gap. She drove for some time around the neighbouring villages before finally deciding the only destination that made sense was her friend Yvonne's house, under a mile away. Yvonne would provide camaraderie and reassurance, and most of all she'd advise her what the hell she should do next for herself and her family.

Our mother wouldn't have been the first woman foolish enough to believe things could change in her marriage. So it was that we returned to an empty cottage later that same night. The broken windows had been boarded over. A truce of some sort had been agreed between our parents on the phone and our father stayed away for a week. His temporary absence provided Mum with space to contemplate our future. But at this point, she condemned our move to the cottage as a complete disaster.

Our father won Mum round. How he convinced her that his supposed affair had been a misunderstanding is in itself proof that miracles do happen.

The truce was uneasy. Jason now had other concerns about the cottage as we listened intently to the voices from the lounge below every evening from our bedrooms. When muffled conversation amplified we held our breath, waiting for an escalation, the danger signs of looming conflict. Jason employed his tatty rag comforter with ardour as we listened attentively until we couldn't fight sleep any longer. Yearned for peace and stability, Jason became increasingly reclusive.

For him, our father was everything and he feared that his leaving forever would mark the end of everything he longed for, someone that might someday reassure him everything would be okay in the end. As the days continued, we began tentatively believing the tide had turned as the knot of angst loosened its grip.

"So why did he finally leave?" Jason stared at our mother unblinking, remembering the empty day he knew his father would never return. The three of us had met to talk things over years later. She explained that a few weeks after 'Rockgate', they'd gone to meet her parents for lunch at The Elephant and Castle. This pub was perched on a short, sharp elevation and was a favourite of ours since the garden contained a play area big enough for us to escape the dark mysterious world of adults and run around carefree. But that weekend we weren't invited. We were dropped at Yvonne's house where Jason watched our parents' car disappear from view with further dejection and fear. Yvonne told my mother that Jason had stared out of the window for half an hour before she could tempt him away.

At the pub, to her dismay it was quickly evident that her parents had invited them for unofficial marriage guidance, everything Mum didn't want. Her parents' marriage was tumultuous at the best of times and they were ill-equipped to offer advice on hers. However, this intervention was through concern for her and their grandchildren so she resigned herself to endure it. Mum could endure anything.

For our father, it would be only the beginning of his discomfort that afternoon. Fearful of upsetting my gangster grandfather – as he perceived him – our father knew he was very much under the microscope. Spending this time with his in-laws was stifling as he glanced repeatedly at his watch, counting the minutes. Was his father-in-law thinking of ways to dispose of him if he didn't convince him he'd look after his daughter in the correct manner?

Yet there was no warning of the unexpected events that unfolded. The father of the young woman our father had been suspected of having an affair with suddenly stormed into the pub wearing a tweed suit and an angry scowl. He took no notice of the company our father had. He had business to discuss and he wasn't going to do it with any civility. Mum says it was like being thrust into a soap opera.

"I want a fucking word with you, you bastard," the man shouted at our father as he marched towards the table. "You've been having it off with my daughter, you dirty bastard." He jabbed his finger at my father's chest.

The age gap was only a minor consideration since she was after all an adult. His true anger was fuelled by a loathing of the number of married men in the area he knew were playing around behind their wives' backs. Mum watched dumbfounded, hating her own naïvety. The drama turned to horror as he lunged, fist back ready to strike, determined to teach our father a lesson.

The rest of the patrons gawped silently, waiting for the gripping finale. The pub was a quintessential country inn where fights were rare and the Sunday regulars observed the spectacle with the same bewilderment as our mother. Leo jumped to his feet and sprinted towards the door. He didn't look back as he ran across the car park. The antique dealer gave chase to no avail as our father roared off down the road in his car. He never lived with us again.

In that brief space of time as my mother stared at the empty space in the car park, the only reminder of my father's presence was his upturned pint glass dripping beer onto the pub floor. A few days later, she discovered through a friend that he'd fled to hook up with this girl and set up a love nest near London. The final remnants of my parents' marriage had vanished.

Jason shook his head tearfully when Mum finished her account, still unable to grasp the finality of this departure despite the passing years.

Later that day, our mother had sat us down and explained that she and our father couldn't live together anymore. It wasn't good for us to hear the fighting.

"Will Dad come back to see us?" Jason had asked fretfully. Mum shrugged disconsolately.

"I'm sure he'll come back and see you." She couldn't look him in the eye though.

Still unsure, he asked me the same thing later that day. He asked this whenever he thought about his father, which for a nine year-old became tiresome, especially on rainy days when the garden was out of reach and we traced the raindrops down the living-room window hoping for a patch of blue to emerge. To my recollection, our father had always been distant, but for Jason there was a different connection I could never understand.

"You used to wait at the bottom of the stairs for Dad if he'd been out drinking, Jason. It used to annoy me."

"I always hoped he'd take notice of me." Jason stared at me unblinking. "I couldn't help it. Some needs you can't explain." He studied the old track marks inside his forearm and on the top of his hands pitifully.

My own conclusion about these events was that nothing had really changed except that Mum was now fretting about money and being able to afford things we'd taken for granted. When she resorted to rationing the tradition of sweets on a Sunday, we understood wholeheartedly that things were heading quickly in the wrong direction.

Several months later Jason and I were told, "Your father's coming to see you tomorrow." Mum said this as if declaring the start of another world war.

Jason's jubilation with this news was to be short-lived. We stood out on the patio that Saturday morning and watched our father's car crawl up the driveway, trying to ignore the surrounding melancholy. But there was to be no happy reunion or hugs for his children.

9

WAS JASON RIGHT?

"Quick. Come inside," Mum shouted, crouching inside the porch one afternoon. Jason and I were racing Matchbox cars around Sean who was sat in the middle of a blanket watching with serene amusement. A car parked at the bottom of the driveway and the doors began opening. "Come inside. Now!" Mum pleaded in a loud whisper, her hands ushering us wildly.

Brutus, the German Shepherd dog my grandfather had given us for protection, barked loudly. Brutus was generally well mannered but when it came to guarding his family he was a fierce protector. Pushing us inside, Mum locked the doors.

"Wait here," she pleaded, pointing to the sofa, "and be quiet." Still crouching, she stooped into the kitchen like a sniper and peered surreptitiously through the windows. Brutus' bark escalated to a loud, violent snarl. The two men standing at the other side of the gate pondered the slim likelihood of getting past fifty kilos of angry canine without injury.

"What's going on?" Jason asked.

"Someone's here Mum doesn't want to see," was my logical explanation.

"Is it Dad?" Jason asked hopefully.

As we sat in the lounge listening, Brutus gradually quietened. Peace returned and we listened to the car coast gently up the lane, stopping parallel to the back gate beside the kitchen.

"Shit," Mum muttered. Crouching, she stared out of the side window with eyes firmly fixed on something the other side of the gate. Brutus began another snarling tirade. Above the din a man's voice attempted to reason.

"We just want to have a chat, Mrs King. That's all we're asking."

Mum turned to us, confused and anxious. We stared back without comprehension as Brutus continued relentlessly.

"Mrs King, if you could just put your dog inside somewhere safe, we need to have a chat," the nervous voice pleaded. Shaking her head and muttering to herself, Mum came back into the lounge.

"Go down into the playroom and be quiet, boys." She pointed to the door by the fireplace.

"Who is it, Mum?" Jason asked fearfully, eyes already red.

"People that want to collect some money, that's all." She tried sounding casual, as if giving people money meant nothing, but as we knew we had none it meant everything. Mum fought tearfully for composure. Back in the kitchen, drained of resolve, she unlocked the back door. "Bru. Come in, Bru." Brutus went quiet, his big paws padded on the kitchen lino then upstairs where my mother locked him safely in her bedroom.

"Is it safe to come in, Mrs. King?" another voice asked from the other side of the gate.

"Come in. I've locked the dog upstairs." Our mother sounded more afraid than ever.

"Mum always dealt with everything on her own, didn't she?" Jason reminisced sadly when we discussed that fateful day. It would be a turning point. In the playroom with the door closed, we'd sat on the sofa opposite the television, Jason anxiously stroking his blanket comforter against his cheek. We watched the closed door apprehensively. Placing my ear against it, I'd vowed that if there were any signs of imminent danger I'd sprint upstairs and release Brutus. Jason crept up and joined me.

It all began to make sense as we discussed our mother's recent stranger than usual behaviour. She would watch the comings and goings of vehicles passing the lane with increasing agitation. Jason always picked up on it first. We were about to learn the truth.

"Mrs King, the mortgage hasn't been paid for many months. We have to serve this Notice of repossession." The silence lingered before Mum began sobbing.

"I've got three kids. My husband's left me with nothing. I need to keep a roof over their heads."

She snivelled as if she'd given up completely. This wasn't like her. She was resourceful, she bought cheap cuts from the butcher to feed us on a pittance; some meals were good, some not so good. If she returned home with a pig's head, we'd fear opening the fridge once she'd prepared this cheap protein. Brawn, a bowl of wobbling mush, filled us with dread. Yet whatever she put in front of us would have to be consumed without objection.

Too stubbornly proud to ask her father for help, Mum's relationship with him was mostly mediocre. By then, she'd understood that her parents didn't want her to stay on in the cottage, believing she was too isolated and vulnerable. Although Sid's business was finally blossoming, Mum believed that if she burdened him financially it would impact on their relationship further. Her only option would be to sell up and rent somewhere she could afford. Now she feared she wouldn't even be able to do that.

"I don't know what I'm going to do." She gazed through the kitchen window hopelessly.

"We're very sorry, Mrs King, really. It's a terrible time for all of you. We hate doing this, you know." The man's voice softened, sounding like a kindly uncle rather than a debt collector.

"Call me Carol," Mum croaked before crying again. The two men conferred for a while.

"Carol, why don't we just leave and pretend we haven't had this conversation today." I heard the click of a briefcase and I imagined the startled look on my mother's face. "It will be several more weeks before any action can be taken anyway. We'll delay things our end as much as possible. But I suggest in the meantime you get a solicitor."

The voices went silent and I heard my mother manage a tearful, "Thank you."

"Good luck, love."

The back door closed and Mum sat crying alone a while longer. As the side gate closed, Brutus began barking again. Finally the door to the playroom opened.

"Good boys. You can come out now."

We followed her into the kitchen where she poured herself a glass of wine. Jason sat beside her, studying her face with concern.

"Are you okay?" he asked, tugging at her sweater.

"It's all going to be fine. But we need to find somewhere else to live. Somewhere nicer that we can afford." She smiled, doing everything she could to muster optimism as we surveyed the kitchen with memories both happy and distressing. Yet Mum would exclaim tearfully on several occasions that we were well and truly in the shit.

From then on, strangers played a bigger part in our lives.

We did receive support. After school, a man from Social Services came and explained to Mum what help she could get. The school gave us free school meals and uniforms.

One Saturday morning, there was a loud knock on the porch door. Brutus flew from under the table barking furiously as my mother glared through the window.

"Can I help you?" she asked, through a gap she'd opened in the window.

"I 'eard you was a bit down on yer luck, sweet'art." The stranger's coarse burr immediately fascinated us as we tried peering out at him.

"Sit down, boys," she demanded, but we couldn't take our eyes off the man with the big sack by the door. "What do you want?" she asked him politely.

The stranger smiled. He looked like a farmer, robust and rugged, hands like hams, testimony to manual toil.

"I have a few 'taters left over and some cabbage I was dropping off for yer. Thought you could use some good 'ome-grown veg."

Mum's face softened into a smile of recognition.

"Didn't you do some work for us a few years ago?"

"That's right. I cleared the pond an' fill it. Did a few other bits and bobs too," the stranger replied.

It struck me as a kind thing to do for someone, making a food donation. The man looked stern but had a good heart. Other strangers would turn up, always an enigma to us, half filling us with fear and half with intrigue.

When Brutus jumped the fence and attacked a passing neighbour's dog, it was a stranger who whisked him away to live on a nearby farm to escape the destruction order. When Mum couldn't afford oil for the heating and hot water, a stranger gave us some of his. Now Dad was gone, strangers became friends – and some friends became strangers.

Our father had now fled to Lincolnshire and the desperately needed maintenance money was never paid. Eventually, our grandfather organised a solicitor and an agreement was reached giving Mum enough time to sell the cottage, pay her debts and be left with just enough to secure a private rental nearby.

Realising another move was imminent, we savoured our last few months enjoying the garden with rejuvenated enthusiasm. The heat of that summer had magically animated the once secretive neighbours inhabiting the cottages along the lane. Like the ants' nest that Jason and I tormented with sticks, the weather seemed to bring everything to life. Our unseen neighbours became sociable, undeniable proof to us that normal life existed after all. It had been rare, during the six years we'd lived there, to see anyone passing our cottage.

It seemed as if all the water in England had dried up completely that summer. Our surrounding countryside transformed into a sweltering brown alien landscape we no longer recognised. The view of the nearby South Downs we still remember as a succession of barren earth mounds baked by the incessant scorching sun. The air was dusted with a bewildering array of insects that annoyed us during the day and tormented us at night, flying forays through the open windows of Fir Tree Cottage.

"You know how much I hated it inside. I was bothered by things I saw and then that summer massive insects came and attacked us." Jason looked pleased with his recollection as I read him another chapter of this book. "You hated stag beetles, didn't you, Marc?" he snorted with amusement, picturing me flying around the bedroom trying to avoid these behemoths. To us they were probably highly venomous transmuted moth bats, sent from Hell at night to terrorise us.

To our dismay there was the added frustration of a hosepipe ban so we had to be especially careful playing our favourite taboo game of drenching each other with water behind the garage lean-to. Jason was a different kid outside, and we were outside all day during that hot summer. As a flower flourishes in sunlight, the summer coaxed Jason from his reclusiveness.

That carefree game was a highlight of the summer, our last summer in the cottage, and my last recollection of my nine year-old brother being truly happy. This was when I began losing sight of my brother. Soon I would realise that Jason had become a stranger.

"Around the age of nine," Jason commented, "I was more aware that the things I sometimes saw maybe weren't normal. I think that's why I'd disappear into my own world – to distract my mind when it worried me." His sudden revelation caused me to pause. It added a piece to the puzzle of what I remembered about my kid brother's increasing detachment.

I also remembered one particular night when I'd begun to wonder whether Jason had been right all along. Perhaps he could indeed see the 'someone' or 'something' he claimed to converse with in his bedroom but which I never saw. These days, he was more inclined to playing alone. With hindsight, I believe that even then I was aware this change wasn't just attributable to growing up. For a while I'd felt envious of the bonhomie he shared with his imaginary friend, and curious whether this was somehow responsible for the shift in our relationship.

When Mum had left for the pub the evening before, it was peaceful in the garden. The birdsong diminished and the blushing summer sky turned crimson behind the Downs, the reddening glow burning behind the fir tree's limbs like a celestial halo. As we watched TV, Jason became quieter. If he wasn't playing with his Action Men or some other toy to absorb his attention his next retreat was always, reluctantly, his bed.

"Will Mum be home soon?" he asked on his way up.

"Yes, soon. When you wake she'll be back. 'Night."

One white lie from time to time was useful if it was what Jason needed as he secured himself under his covers. As the older brother, I was responsible for nullifying his fears on the rare occasions we were left alone. Babysitters were a rarity and expensive. The nearest one lived on the outskirts of the village, only available when she wasn't studying, and we barely knew any of our neighbours well enough. Restless and sensitive, Jason stroked his face with his comforter as I watch his anxious eyes from the end of my bed. Our sixteen-month age gap felt much greater during these moments.

We felt isolated when Mum went to meet friends at night. Sean was easy, once asleep he never woke. But Jason often stared at the blackness on the other side of the empty room. Whenever I asked what he was looking at or who he was talking to he'd shake his head and tell me he was just playing.

Once my brothers were asleep that night, fear tiptoed in. I lay in bed rocking, wishing away the night and hoping for the familiar rumble of Mum's car crunching the gravel driveway. Looking after my brothers empowered me with a superficial bravery but now I felt restless with angst. The room was hot and sticky. The path beyond Jason's window that by day was a treasured secret route became a mysterious dark underworld at night.

I began humming to one of the records we'd heard Mum crying to as she played it over and over. I rocked and hummed with my fingers in my ears to blot out all sound. It helped pass the time and distract my mind from other things I was beginning to imagine.

The cottage wasn't old, it just behaved like it was, creaking and groaning, always harbouring unexplainable melancholy. Its sounds bothered us, they weren't the natural night sounds from outside that we knew. Owls and foxes could be disconcerting but they were familiar, organic.

Unable to sleep and becoming too exhausted to rock, I released my fingers and listened to hollow nothingness. Then I gradually became aware within the stillness of sounds I didn't like, sounds that sent my thoughts haywire: a clang of the fireplace tools disturbed by a mischievous breeze from the chimney, a creaking door or floorboard. Cups clinking in the kitchen would trick me into believing Mum was home. Listening harder to extraneous noises heightened my anxiety. I couldn't ignore the sounds and they became an obsession. A squeak became the latch to the stairway doors opening and an avalanche of irrational thoughts.

I persuaded myself to open my eyes. I'd left the bulb above the stairwell on and I focused on the light filtering through the sizeable gap at the bottom of the door, hoping not to see a passing shadow of footsteps on the landing. The noises and bumps were there, keeping me teetering precariously on the edge of panic.

"You awake, Jason?" I uttered into the blackness behind the banisters, half-hoping that he was, half-hoping he'd remain within his oblivious security.

The resounding silence was making me feel abandoned. Reluctantly, I gazed into the darkness outside my window, wishing Mum home so I could endure the cottage with bravery again. The only thing visible with my chin resting hesitantly on the windowsill was the black void of the lean-to, sending a rush of dejection through me like a spear. I prayed to hear popping stones and a rumbling engine.

Forcing my head back onto the pillow, upset by my inability to control the anxiety, I really began panicking. Nothing would pacify me. I thought about phoning someone. But whom? No family lived nearby. And where would I find any numbers anyway? There was no-one. I considered running into the night to the only neighbour we knew, but even Roy was a relative stranger whose cottage was at the bottom of an adjoining misty and winding lane. Then what would I say, what had forced me into the night, abandoning my brothers? I pictured his weathered face in the dark seclusion of his cottage.

I heard a thud downstairs and wished we still had Brutus, my heart pounding in my ears like a drum. I suddenly sat bolt upright, sweat running down my face and back.

Then there was the droning grumble of a car popping stones as it entered our lane. With unreserved relief, I leaned out of the window watching the headlights enter the lean-to. Like a morphine shot, calmness returned. The engine ran for a while, the lights still on. I urgently wanted Mum to turn off the engine and come inside. I wanted to hear the porch door and front door closing, then finally the stairway doors. Then I'd feel safe.

Through the darkness I watched Mum leaning on the car, trying to lock it, swaying slightly before finally walking slowly across the gravel. Just before the patio steps she stopped abruptly. She was almost below my window. I could sense her bewilderment. Mum looked up into the night air as though smelling it, aware of something. I couldn't hear anything apart from the drumming in my ears.

She pirouetted awkwardly to face the lean-to again. Had she forgotten her cigarettes or purse? As she paused on the bottom step, a deep heavy thud slammed against the corrugated plastic roof of the garage. The sound made us both jump. Mum sprinted up the remaining steps, terrified. Her keys jangled desperately as she fumbled with the lock then the slamming porch door sent a shockwave through the cottage. Miraculously, Jason and Sean remained asleep. By the time I'd reached my bedroom door, Mum was urgently closing the door to the stairs behind her. She looked up at me startled and fearful.

"Come here," she instructed breathlessly.

Yanking me into her room by my arm she pushed me towards her bed, switched off the lights, kicked off her shoes and flung her jacket behind her. Jumping into bed, she pulled me in beside her. Her fear was tangible, renewing mine.

In the total darkness we listened to footsteps outside the window, heavy and purposeful. I still remember them clearly, swift, decisive and almost theatrical. The footsteps travelled from the front of the cottage towards her room at the back then stopped suddenly. From my intimate knowledge of every inch of the garden, they'd stopped beside the back door to the kitchen. The ensuing silence became deafening. We were both listening, hearts banging, not daring to utter a syllable, hoping our silence would make us undetectable. But from what?

"Marc, look through the curtains. See who it is," Mum hissed desperately into my ear. I didn't want to go, any more than I wanted to be in the house with my brothers when she had gone out. Yet I wanted her to know I was the man of the house and that thought gave me the fortitude I needed. Fearfully tiptoeing across the floor, I waited breathless just behind the curtains as Mum huddled behind the covers.

"Look. Just take a quick look," she pleaded.

My hands warily found a gap. In the warmth of that balmy summer night, I felt cold and nauseous. I carefully pulled the curtain aside just enough to observe the blackness, the emptiness tinged with the eerie light between night and dawn. There was nothing. The back door of the kitchen was closed, the garden was empty, and soon the familiar contours of trees and shrubs would become visible again. My anxiety eased.

"There's no-one, Mum," I murmured, relieved.

She beckoned me back to bed and I climbed beside her gladly. Sighing, she held me with such intensity I struggled for breath. I could feel and hear the wild rhythm of her heart. The lingering familiar scent of a happy night out, the fags, booze and faded perfume, comforted me to sleep.

In the morning I woke up in our mother's bed, fixing my gaze upon the gap in the curtains, listening to the first welcome birdsong. The same gap where I'd stood transfixed by fear in the early hours of that morning. My mother was still asleep, the room permeated with the bittersweet scent of her previous night's excesses at The Queen's Head. I didn't wake her. She deserved to extract any happiness she could from life. Although we hated being left alone at night, I was happy to see her gain respite from her depression.

At eleven, I was beginning to be more thoughtful and to question things manfully. For example, I knew that adults say one thing when they nearly always mean another. Like when Mum reassured Jason, "Of course your father wants to see you, he's just very busy", I understood perfectly that no father is too busy for two years. So now I reassured myself that I hadn't seen anything threatening in the darkness last night.

Yet we'd both heard it.

After that experience, I thought about Jason's strangeness more and more over the next few weeks as his mood diminished further.

10

LEAVING THE GREEN PLACE

In a small woodland, a short leafy walk from the cottage, Jason made a rare appearance from his increasing solitude. Along with his friend Martin, they put the finishing touches to the dam they'd constructed. The woods here were a regular retreat for neighbourhood kids. It was the pattern of the countryside we lived in, small lanes and roads dissecting rural playgrounds in which we explored our imagination.

Meticulously, they'd successfully blocked the passage of the stream running through the bed of the woods. Jason straddled the trickling water leaking from a gap, using his hands like a crane as Martin passed sticks and moss. Placing the detritus carefully, Jason plugged the leak.

"It's finished." He beamed triumphantly, the dimples in his cheeks like tiny grinning craters. It was always a triumph whenever my happy brother returned. "Let's watch the dam overflow and flood the kingdom."

Jason's playfulness gained momentum as he gazed down at the stream and imaginary kingdom he'd created. All I could see was a succession of sticks, stones and rocks. But to Jason the sticks marked the kingdom's boundaries, the small stones and rocks he'd gathered represented its people and buildings respectively. He sat observing the rising floodwater. I was mesmerised, caught in the web of his infectious ability to make me believe in the games he'd conceive and direct, in enchanted lands and the mythical creatures within. I envied his talent. From my frequent apathy he triggered avid fascination.

The upper level of the swelling stream matured into a small rising lake quickly reaching the rim of the dam.

"Run! Run! It's going to burst." Jason plucked the sticks and stones from the soft mud. Somewhere in the branches of a nearby tree a cuckoo sounded the alert. The water cascaded over the sticks and moss and flooded my brother's kingdom. Jason threw a lichen-covered stick into the water and watched the spreading ripples.

"We're leaving our cottage." He glanced at Martin dismally.

"We'll still be nearby though, Jason," I reminded him, hoping to ease his dismay.

"We haven't got any money," Jason explained.

"Will you still be able to come to the woods?" Martin asked.

Jason shrugged, looking down at the broken dam, and I sensed his realisation that at some point or another in life there was an end to everything. My brother craved security, something to provide consistency for him, a stable home especially, and he felt the effects of change far more than me.

Mum searched for somewhere local to rent so we could attend the same schools. A solicitor crunched the numbers and calculated that once the main debts were paid, there should be enough equity from the sale of the cottage to release funds to last her a year, perhaps more.

Although Sid wanted his daughter to live nearer, she again stubbornly refused his offer. Being a hard-nosed businessman who'd never received a leg up in his life, Sid believed his daughter when she insisted she could manage alone. If Mum could harvest anything from the shambolic move to the cottage, it would surely be her pride. She figured that, even if she failed, at least she'd earn respect for trying. If she let Sid take the reins, she knew she'd be granting him bragging rights at the golf club. She could almost see the admiration in the clubhouse as her father boasted to his drinking cronies about his endless benevolence.

"How long before we leave?" Jason asked one bedtime.

"We won't be leaving for quite a while," Mum informed him before briskly leaving the room.

Her answer had been unsatisfactory for both of us. Again the mysterious narrative concerning timings that adults used was confounding.

"How long is quite a while?" Jason's inquisition began earnestly once she'd left. "Is it longer than two weeks?"

"Yes. I think it's longer than three or four weeks even." In the darkness I could almost hear my brother's next question forming.

"Will we move before Christmas?" The bedsprings twanged as Jason shifted position. "Will we be going to the same schools?" He fired his questions up through the darkness. Frustrated, I ran out of patience.

"I don't know, Jason," I snapped, aware I'd failed to live up to his expectation of being the oracle of all knowledge. "Sorry, Jason. We'll have to wait and see."

It was actually six weeks before we moved, from a mysterious cottage with a magical garden to a flat above a butcher's and a hardware store. Mum initially felt pleased she'd found and secured the flat. It was conveniently situated in an area of the village near the bus stop where the coach took us to our respective schools.

"You know, there have only been three places I've lived where I haven't seen or experienced anything weird. The flat was one of them," Jason told me later, as if having an epiphany. "But even though I never experienced anything inside the flat, I'd sometimes see things I didn't understand outside, like strangers who seemed out of place. It's difficult to explain unless you saw them like me."

I often think about this. If Jason was traumatised by changes and strangeness, then the more he would feel compelled to find a solution, something that could provide connection, stability and perhaps even obliteration.

Our new garden was a stunted patch of uneven turf making

simple tasks like passing a football impossible as it would ricochet off the lunar landscape and disappear into the knotted rhododendrons. On the other side of the garden was the wall of the newsagent who, we quickly discovered, didn't appreciate the slap of a football every few seconds. We were mostly confined inside and the outside wasn't much better.

The flat ran the entire length of the shops beneath and although the living space was adequate it wasn't homely, just somewhere to sleep, eat and wash. It didn't possess that unquantifiable air of edginess that existed at Fir Tree Cottage which, I soon discovered, I missed terribly. The flat was bland. During the previous six years, we'd somehow grown accustomed to living in a home that was an unexplainable mystery.

On the other hand, blowing cigarette smoke across our dingy downstairs kitchen each morning, Mum looked relieved to no longer have the burden of the cottage around her neck. She believed she could manage the flat alone. For the first time in years, she alone was in control of our destiny.

I'd started at the grammar school ten miles away while Jason remained at the nearer intermediate school and Sean at the infant school in the village. Although more settled, though, Jason was becoming increasingly reclusive. Our Uncle Reg overheard us discussing friendships one day.

"In your entire lifetime, you can count your true friends on one hand," he told us. "They're the friends to cherish." It became a quote Jason relished, giving an order of normality to his solitary lifestyle. Finding that handful of true friends had always been and would remain a challenge.

We faced other new challenges after the move. I returned home each day feeling miserable and out of place at school.

"I don't like my new school, Jace," I remember telling him despondently one afternoon, slumping on the sofa like a sack of potatoes. Despite Jason's increased solitude, our respective roles unexpectedly reversed.

"It'll just take time to get used to, Marc," he offered astutely, conscious of my unhappiness. I considered him with awe as he continued appraising his Action Man apparel laid out on the living room carpet for the third time since I'd got home. He looked up and smiled. "Everything will turn out okay in the end," he assured me. Whilst I loved his kindness, I couldn't fathom where this profound wisdom had come from.

Indeed, we became troubled kinsmen, he no longer just my younger brother but a friend who'd try his best to offer counsel despite his increasing pursuit of solitude. Always sympathetic and ready to listen, Jason became my stress ball. He relished this new status, as if my anxieties provided a welcome distraction from his own unspoken challenges.

He placed his new Stretch Armstrong next to two Action Men, drawing the number three on a piece of paper.

"Why do you always do everything in threes?" I asked.

"I just like to. I can't help it," he shrugged.

Struggling with new quirks he didn't understand, Jason was still happy to exist anywhere where Mum was all right. Without the millstone of the cottage, she became calmer and happier and he enjoyed a brief unsteady period of serenity.

The flat inflicted fresh restrictions, though. If we played with too much enthusiasm, Mum received complaints about the noise from the shopkeepers below and a warning from the landlord. The no-noise rule was enforced rigidly. We considered this an infringement of our liberty, Jason less so as he was always content to be alone in his room.

I felt indignant about this hanging threat of eviction and went looking for mischief, trespassing into newly built houses and breaking into the sheds of local residents. My brief experimentation with a life of crime caused bemusement for Jason on the numerous occasions the local policeman came to caution me. Jason remembers his concerns of that time.

"If you'd been sent to Reform School, Marc, I'd have felt even more alone."

As we got older, our mother shared her daily struggles readily, which only concerned Jason even more. She'd always been good with money but this new perspective made us realise how difficult things were, still dealing with debts on top of our daily needs of food and warmth. The flat was to be our long-term home and, although it was far from perfect, we were all determined to make the most of it.

A few months after the move, I came home from school to an awkward atmosphere. Jason and Sean were sitting at the table bench in the kitchen with Mum on the opposite side. My silent brothers wore confused expressions, Jason's bordering on fear. I said hello to everyone and Mum cleared her throat as if about to make a speech.

Only then did I notice someone else sitting at the table. Staring from the darkest corner was a bearded stranger with unkempt hair. Jason and I later agreed that at first glance he looked like a mixture of Jesus as depicted on the windows of the local church and a festival hippy.

"Animal is going to be our lodger." Mum spoke about this figure with fond familiarity as though we already knew him. Animal? I looked at Jason's confused expression and realised I'd been foolish to think things could be normal for too long. I knew from friends what normality looked like, and the mad grinning hippy opposite wasn't it. He beamed with an inane smirk and wild beady eyes, trying his best to appear like a friendly uncle.

"What's a lodger?" Jason beat me to the golden question.

"Someone who helps pay the bills." Mum and Animal began laughing and then the answer dawned on me, watching Animal's shoulder spasms, his wild eyes peering through his excessive head and facial hair.

"I get it. Animal. Like the Muppet character?"

"You got it, light bulb." He pointed a chubby digit towards me with a grin. As absurd as the moment was, my brothers and I found his laughter infectious, tickled by the sight of his bobbing head throwing wayward strands of flailing hair around.

Animal was sometimes a welcome distraction as well as a

source of intrigue for the three of us. Educated, articulate and extremely eccentric, he possessed the traits required to keep three inquisitive young minds transfixed. Jason in particular found our lodger fascinating and, without knowing it, Animal temporarily drew him from his increasing solitude.

Sean moved into Jason's room, leaving the lodger his bedroom which, within a few weeks, became an eclectic dumping ground for his curious belongings. Camera bodies hung from the window handles, lenses were lined up on the windowsill, books and magazines were strewn across the floor as if it had been struck by a miniature tornado. More substantial publications were stacked on the bedside cabinet, the only other furniture in the room, and piles of his clothes filled every corner. We'd peruse the manic disorder with fascination.

"Now, I wonder what shirt I'll wear today?" He'd stand by his bed in a pair of shorts and fetid tee-shirt, hunching over a clothes pile like a hairy spider.

"You're mad," Jason would declare, laughing as the bedroom door slammed and then almost immediately reopened to reveal Animal in cheesecloth shirt and faded denim flairs.

In providing bizarre platonic companionship for Mum, our lodger could be kind. But he could also be spiteful when his playfulness got out of hand. We grew accustomed to the occasional unexpected dead leg while watching TV, and seeing Jason retreat to his room to cry without shame was more painful than enduring my own pain. We'd often sit together there, watching the throbbing red patches in the centre of our thighs with anger.

"Remember when Animal threw you in the rhododendrons?" Jason commented with amusement when we reminisced.

It was during a game of football that Animal grew bored of retrieving the ball from the hedge. Dropping the ball, he grabbed me and pushed me up above his head, then launched me into the rhododendrons. My horror at realising I was no longer in his grip but travelling towards the spiteful branches was tangible. My crash through the undergrowth was followed by the pandemonium of snapping twigs and agony as branches bit through my tee-shirt and into my flesh.

"You okay, Marc? Should I get Mum?" As Jason pulled me from the vegetation, I considered the ramifications, the loss of income and camaraderie for her.

"I'm okay." I bit my lip, feeling hurt and angry.

"That... was... dangerous!" My kid brother berated Animal, mustering something close to fury despite his timidity. We limped back to the confines of my bedroom where, with Jason as witness, I allowed a trickle of tears to betray my humiliation.

"I think that episode confirmed our suspicions, Jace," I muttered. "He really was an animal and best avoided."

A year after moving into the flat, fate presented our family with another unkind twist. Slamming the phone down one afternoon, Mum told the caller to "Go fuck yourself. I'm not paying it." She sat dejectedly on the sofa. It turned out that the landlord was insisting the absurdly high electricity bills she'd disputed for months were her responsibility; some obscure clause in the small print on the lease meant that Mum was liable not only for our electricity but also for that of the shops below. It was a push too far. We couldn't afford to live there anymore.

So it was that one Saturday morning several weeks later, a friend of hers arrived at the flat with a removals van. The only prior warning of this had been the previous evening. Waiting until we were settled in front of the TV, Mum instructed us to start packing our belongings into the boxes she'd been accumulating. To wreak the perfect revenge upon the unjust landlord, she'd planned this clandestine move without telling a soul. The landlord would be the last person to discover we'd done a runner, once he'd forced his way into the flat to find mess, emptiness and the neatly stacked pile of final demands. Meanwhile, we headed back to our grandparents' bungalow.

"How long are we going to live back at Grandad's?" Jason asked anxiously. We watched her expectantly, giddy with her second revelation that we'd soon be leaving Sussex for good, once she'd found a house and schools. We'd be moving nearer to our other grandparents in south-west London. Mum had swallowed her pride and allowed her father to help, believing she was doing the right thing in the long term for her family.

Jason became quieter, contemplating two moves in succession with solitary trepidation. In the event, it took another year.

We'd grown to love the countryside, which had become our best friend and comforter, and now we were leaving the green place for good. We accepted it with trepidation as Jason took a further nosedive and the connection between us became more remote and often hard to bridge. He became more reclusive and inclined to disappear into make-believe worlds as he struggled to cope with another change. As our belongings stored in the garage decayed with the damp, if felt as though our friendships did the same, that by saying goodbye we were bidding farewell to friendships entirely.

"I felt like we were moving country, not county," Jason remarked disconsolately one afternoon.

When we visited the big school in London before the end of the summer term, it felt austere and imposing. The frenetic order in the playground seemed cold and uncaring as the Headmaster guided us around like the new school pets. When we left that afternoon, we felt insignificant. And by the end of our first year, Jason had completed his reverse metamorphosis, becoming as insular as a chrysalis. One reason became clear when he arrived at the bus stop for our journey home pale and depressed, without his glasses.

"Where are your glasses?" I asked. He pulled them from his pocket, one arm snapped and one lens missing.

"I stuck them together with Sellotape but they broke again during PE," he informed me miserably.

"How did they get broken?"

"Bullies." My brother looked at the pavement shaking his head, tears streaming. I sat on the bus fuming, while Jason stared through the window, lost in another world. Our mother flew into a rage at the school for allowing this.

Liked by everyone who got to know him, Jason remained on the fringe of school friendships and few others spent time with him after school. Struggling to integrate, he became more vulnerable to other influences.

One day, as I read a draft of this chapter and we discussed this move, Jason suddenly brightened with another recollection.

"Do you remember Sean's toy spaceship that turned itself on in our room?"

"I remember the big argument that followed when you accused him of turning it on," I replied. Jason grinned, his tarnished teeth witness to a life of regrets.

"And Mum had a go at me for taking down the horse brasses as well, remember?" he continued. I waited patiently, wondering where this would lead. This often happened when we discussed childhood.

"It was just after she'd got the house sorted after the move. I went downstairs one morning and all her horse brasses were on the lounge floor in a perfect line. That's when I realised that something must have followed me from the cottage. She accused me of taking them down but I told her they were already down. She went mad at me." His hurt was still tangible. "I was eleven, and only this tall." He placed his hand just under his chest. "How could I reach nearly up to the ceiling without a fucking ladder?" Taking another gulp of black coffee he continued, "I'm telling you the truth, Marc. Something followed me."

It was sometimes impossible not to feel irritated with him. I questioned whether I wasn't helping but hindering his mental health by reading these chapters to him.

"Not this again. That's just your messed up mind telling you that. You're hardly ever straight enough to know what reality is."

"Well, I'm straight now," he glared at me, his emotions brimming. "I've not had anything for days. I know I'm telling the truth, Marc." Jason looked betrayed, regretting everything he'd ever confided to me.

That afternoon we continued our conversation about childhood, recalling the kaleidoscope he'd play with in his bedroom. I'd sometimes look through it and be bored within a minute, wondering what the big deal was with those strange hypnotic patterns of symmetry. Whereas Jason could easily spend two hours pointing the lens out of the window, twisting it and ignoring me.

"I'd see more than pretty patterns." Jason gave a wry frown, retrieved the vape I'd bought him for Christmas from his pocket and inhaled, disappearing behind a thick plume of strawberry scented smoke that filled the room. "That kaleidoscope would bring the orbs outside my window. I made the patterns, then the orbs would float across the lens. When I took the kaleidoscope away they'd hover above the garage roof."

Whatever he told me he saw I have to believe. It was his reality. I couldn't doubt Jason's conviction as he stared at me stone-faced, telling his stories.

"When I was older, maybe about eleven, that's when I knew that what I'd seen on that first day at the cottage – the old man by the fireplace – was something paranormal. And I needed to find my own way of stopping it happening again. I've told you, Marc. It's not the drugs. Not all of it. These things are real." Jason looked at the patterns of the carpet, shaking his head.

Then I remembered I had a story that might help ease his dejection. It was something our mother had told me only recently. She had paused in our conversation and looked thoughtfully through the window that afternoon, knitting together the details of something that had apparently mystified her.

A year before leaving the cottage, her friend Pat had dropped her youngest daughter Lucy off to stay for the day. Lucy was a similar age to Sean, about five, also small and cute which made Sean jealous of the attention she commanded, as Mum recalled with her syrupy Silk Cut laugh. Her eyes still fixed somewhere above the hedge outside, Mum's expression became one of absolute concentration.

"Well, Pat's mother Bobby came to collect Lucy later that afternoon. She'd never visited the cottage before but we'd been introduced in The Queen's Head when they moved down to the area a few years before we left the cottage. That's how I met her daughter Pat who was a similar age to me. We all became good friends."

It was satisfying to watch my mother engrossed in the past, as she was becoming progressively disenchanted about the present and future. She was clearly relishing this snapshot memory.

"I'm certain it was springtime. You were all playing outside on the front lawn on a big blanket and I kept my eye on you through the kitchen window. This car came up the driveway and stopped halfway. I thought it had come up by mistake. It then drove further up and parked. Bobby climbed out and walked towards you all.

"She chatted to you and seemed cheerful and I called out to her to come through to the kitchen for a coffee. It took a while before she came through. And then she was strangely quiet and looked shocked." Mum nodded to herself, confirming the details. "Then, out of the blue, she asked me the strangest question. 'Are you okay here, Carol?' It shocked me, why she was asking and looking so serious." Mum paused again, frowned and took another drag on her cigarette.

"I asked her why? I must have looked really surprised. Then Bobby apologised and told me that as she'd walked into the lounge she thought she'd seen someone standing in the corner by the fireplace. I remember I started shaking, thinking no, not this again."

Mum knew she had never discussed the exorcism stuff afterwards and was certain Bobby knew nothing about it.

"It was nearly five years later by this time. We wanted everything forgotten in case we had to sell." She rolled her eyes at the irony.

At the time of Bobby's revelation, our mother was counting

down the days to leaving. The repossession order was being processed and she was searching for a new home to rent. She'd learned not to dwell on the strange stuff that had happened, that was apparently still happening. She panicked about how she'd cope if things nosedived any further for her.

Why this story had remained hidden for so long was a mystery. Perhaps I'd liberated her memory by telling her I was writing about Jason and our time in the cottage.

11

THE BEGINNING
OF THE AFFAIR

"Come round later, Marc, and we can talk about it."

My brother's delight about me visiting his place was always touching. This was his story I was telling, he was the one I was still trying to fathom, like a human Rubik's Cube. Knocking on his door, two apprehensions arose in my mind. The first, of course, was which brother would I find on the other side – the undone madman or the affable, sorry human who was my true brother, the man I wanted to help? Two locks clicked and Jason appeared in the doorway.

"Hello, brother. Come in," Jason beamed. Inside, he leaned over to switch the TV off. One of his favourite channels had been showing, specialising in his less destructive pastime of watching alien documentaries and conspiracy theories as well as outlandish natural history programmes about rare species. Jason could watch for eternity anything with a vaguely abnormal theme.

"You kept your word then, Jace? You seem pretty straight this evening." I patted his shoulder.

"Told you I would, Marc. I'm a man of my word, you should know that by now." Jason snorted a laugh, his shoulders bouncing happily. It was definitely the affable brother I had for company tonight.

My second anxiety was always which chair to sit on. The choice was the splintered wicker two-seater with the bulging seat cushion about to collapse or the once green fabric armchair with the ripped arms littered with cigarette burns and stains that I didn't want to think about. Jason as always, slumped into his favourite beige leather armchair that partially blocked the kitchen entrance. As he sank further into the dishevelled folds of worn, cracked leather, he blended in like a chameleon. I decided there was less anxiety in opting for the stains.

"Marc?" There was a familiar, uncomfortable pause. "Would you mind if I have a little pipe before we start? Helps clear my mind." He wasn't talking Golden Virginia and a pair of paisley slippers. I looked across and shook my head.

"No way, Jason. I know you like your evening hit but you promised to be completely straight. There's some points I want to tidy up so no coke, please."

"You're right, Marc. I need to cut down more." He slumped further into his armchair, nodding in reluctant agreement before snorting self-deprecatingly and retrieving his trusty vape. "I've always needed to cut down."

When we'd met the previous week, we'd begun discussing the beginnings of his drug experiments, that illusive period of his personal history that had escaped me, a preoccupied older teenager. He began telling me of the night, aged sixteen and still living at Mum's house in south London. He'd sat outside The Southampton pub on a grubby bench, sipping a bottle of Special Brew. That early Saturday evening was to be the start of his true decent into narcotics.

The pub is long gone now but every time I look at the office block and shops now occupying the space I think of my brother. He loved the place. It was where his few mates frequented.

"I got chatting to this girl. I couldn't believe my luck." Jason shook his head and his eyes sparkled at the memory. "She seemed to really like me and said she'd seen me about a few times and wanted to talk to me. She was quite a bit older, early twenties.

She asked me if I wanted a drink so I said yes and continued to chat her up. I almost had to pinch myself."

Jason's face burst into a crinkled smile. For some reason thinking about that short affair, as it turned out to be, still brought him happiness as well as regret. Another strange facet of his personality was that he was wary around men and felt happier in the company of women. They took the half hour bus journey back to her house.

"You know what happened next." Jason raised his eyes taking a hard tug on his vape. Later that evening Linda woke with a sudden urge. "She said she needed to go back to the pub and find her brother, Dave. He always held a lot of brown or white, she said. I'd never met him before." Jason shook his head, blowing a plume of smoke at his feet. "It was about ten when we got back. She went inside and came out two minutes later with a wrap of brown."

"Heroin?"

"Yes, Marc." Jason laughed jokily. "I knew I wanted to try it. We went back to hers and I had my first chase on a sheet of foil, my first real high. I just asked her if I could try some and she said 'Of course.' I'd already told her I liked smoking a bit of dope. I remember you told me you'd tried it and didn't like it but I loved it when I first tried it at fourteen. It made me feel good, calm and relaxed."

Jason was displaying mixed emotions at the memory. Suddenly he stood up and reached toward the front door key, flicking the latch lock and turning the key in the second lock before slumping back in his chair.

"It's true what they say, though. For me, dope was a gateway drug. I loved the feeling but wanted something stronger that gave me that freedom for longer."

"Do you still remember that first hit?"

"Like it was yesterday. It was beautiful. It was what I'd been looking for. The Floyd had it spot on, comfortably numb was how I felt." His tranquil frown told me he understood that it was both the best and the worst thing he'd ever inflicted upon himself. "I was flattered that an older women fancied me, Marc. We carried on seeing each other for a while. Eventually I bought a quarter from her for fifteen quid. It was normally twenty-five then but she did me a special discount."

It sounded too good to be true and, sure enough, probing him further about his relationship with Linda I revealed the uncomfortable truth.

"One night in The Southampton she introduced me to her brother, Dave. He'd done time for armed robbery apparently, so Linda told me." Jason raised his eyebrows woefully. "Linda introduced me at the bar and at first it looked like he wanted to kill me. He was a stocky fucker, big scar on his forehead and he just stared at me like he was weighing me up. I thought why the fuck does he want to beat up a skinny sixteen year-old kid?" The fear Jason felt during that first meeting with Dave the robber many years ago was still evident. "Anyway I had my friends there, didn't I? They liked me and I knew I could rely on them if he kicked off."

Jason's like-minded friends in The Southampton were always fond of him. I attributed some of this to his generosity with the dope he held as he'd explained previously, a pinch here and there to keep them happy and friendly. Sometimes to make a bit of extra cash he'd save and buy a half or full ounce and then split it into eighths to make a little extra. This was the start of a regular format for subsidising his habit.

"How old was this Dave, Jason?"

"He was older than Linda, late twenties, maybe thirty? Linda told me to go and sit down and I remember feeling pretty nervous about what was going to happen. Eventually he came over, put his arm around my shoulder and slid a pint of lager in front of me. He said he didn't normally like blokes but he liked me." Jason grinned with satisfaction. That was all my brother ever really wanted throughout his troubled life, to be liked, and he didn't really care by whom, especially at that impressionable age. "He told me not to tell anyone he was selling me gear."

"Why was that?"

"People liked me down The Southampton, didn't they, they'd have sorted him out if they knew he was selling smack to a sixteen year-old." Jason swaggered in his chair but his confidence in his friends was misplaced. I doubted they'd actually give a damn. The ones I met were older men and women with their own obvious needs and troubles.

"So Dave became your dealer, then?" I shook my head thinking of my quiet, sensitive brother's beginnings of surrender to addiction, with friends helping him with discounted rates, perhaps sex and flattery. Once the need was established, a regular supply was made seamlessly accessible.

"So Dave introduced me to Paul who became my mate and used to come to Mum's house every Friday. I'd meet him outside to collect my fix. I was still only smoking it, up in my bedroom." Jason looked at the door again, slightly agitated.

"You know what? You were ahead of your time, Jace." He looked at me confused. "Well before apps were invented you were getting drugs delivered to your door. You could have called it Smackeroo and made a packet."

"Yeah, I was always ahead of my time, Marc." Jason beamed at my ludicrous suggestion. "You know, I was the youngest regular at The Southampton?" He looked triumphant as he sucked his vape and gave me a smoky grin. "But I did my research, you know, Marc. Before taking any drugs. I'm not totally stupid."

"Research? How?"

"The library. We were members, remember? Remember me telling you that's how I found books on drugs, LSD, dope, heroin, everything I needed to know about and wanted to try."

Why was my brother smiling with such a self-satisfied grin?

It wasn't the fault of the librarian who directed Jason's inquisitive mind. Nor was it the fault of the library for containing the information, the menu my brother wanted to work his way through. My brother set his own agenda since discovering a way to calm his turmoil, tame his visions or perhaps find an excuse for them. Most of all, he'd found a friend to tame his loneliness.

"I tried it all but just knew I wanted to take heroin. It was the most efficient way to tranquility, to get away from everything." Yet was it not also, I thought, the most efficient way of making his mental illness worse?

"So anyway, you said you were selling a bit of dope to fund your habit?"

"Just a bit and then I'd get it on tick. Although I never gave tick to anyone," Jason declared breezily, proud of his business acumen as if he were the pub's answer to Alan Sugar. "I quickly discovered dope worked a bit but brown was the best. Stops everything instantly and lasts for hours and hours. If you do it right it can last days before you have to suffer the comedown."

Jason continued developing his taste for the brown over the following six months until the inevitable happened. When he described the scene it brought tears to my eyes, despite my knowing about all his years of using. All I saw was a scared sixteen year-old kid, sensitive to everyone.

"Dave came up to me one Friday night and put a half pint in front of me. He still used to scare me. Then he whispered in my ear, 'D'yer fancy a proper hit?' I said yes immediately."

It was only now that Jason began to show remorse about his habit despite his lingering memories of sweet oblivion, of friendships beginning and of what he sometimes fondly thought of as 'the good times'.

"So where did you go? Not the pub toilets?"

"You know the quiet residential roads around there, Marc? Dave had a minivan, with no windows in the back." Jason laughed in disbelief. "He got all nasty again when we got into the back of the van and told me, 'You know that if you go over I'll have to dump your body?' I hoped he was joking but he didn't even look at me, just started preparing his works." Jason gazed blankly at the mute TV as if watching the scene play out again.

Dave proceeded to cook up a sprinkle of brown with some

water and a bit of lemon juice as a garnish.

"You ready, Jace?"

"I'd already rolled my sleeve up, hungry for it, and used a thin piece of cord tied around the top of my forearm. It was easy to find a good vein. I said, 'Go on, hit me.'"

Dave had slid the needle into the bulging vein and Jason sat for fifteen minutes in tranquility. It spread over him like a cashmere blanket; he was more happy and content than he could ever remember being. He knew then he'd never be alone. He had a friend for life.

I wished I'd been there walking down that tree-lined avenue. I found myself fantasising about what I'd have done to stop this beginning of Jason's dependency. Drag Dave from the car and beat him until he was no more? But it wouldn't have stopped Jason. My brother knew he wanted to find a way out from his reality, his depression and the visitations that harangued him. The only way that moment in his life could have been avoided would have been if his decline had been recognised sooner. By me, for instance.

"We sat in his van for fifteen minutes and then Dave said he could drop me in town as he had some business to do." Jason pulled out a small plastic brown bottle and laughed as he poured a handful of assorted pills into his palm. "This is my suicide kit. There's everything here, Pregabalin, Valium, sleepers and strong painkillers." He popped two Valium into his mouth and swallowed them without water.

"How long did that first hit last, Jace?"

"About three hours or so for the real sensation. I just walked around town in a happy haze without a care about anything. I felt fantastic, like nothing could touch me." He turned his palms up and gazed at the ceiling, like an evangelist giving his testimony. "The comedown was something I'd read and heard about but wasn't fully expecting. That's the worst thing about getting so high, you have to come back down with a bump."

Jason described how he woke up the following morning

early, already feeling irritable and anxious. He knew what would happen next, where he would need to go in a few more hours in order to make him feel the way he had the previous evening.

"After six months of injecting I was doing two or sometimes even ten hits a day at weekends." His habit had been truly established well before his seventeenth birthday, with the careful influence of others. "I found as long as I only did a bit at a time I could carry on fairly normally. But then I found other things to experiment with. When I started doing speedballs I found out I could drink anyone under the table." His eyes widened still in disbelief at his former powers.

"What's a speedball exactly?"

"Cocaine, heroin, speed and sometimes some prescription opiates if the smack is shit. I used to shoot them up, had the first one on my seventeenth birthday."

I sighed with sorrow. Jason had never before completely divulged the chronology of his early addiction. In one session, he claimed to have drunk a school rugby player we knew under the table. Despite being tall and gangly, Jason possessed mind-bending resilience. My brother was so ashamed of his skinny legs he'd insist on wearing Long Johns under his trousers to give his legs more bulk, even in the summer. The drugs enhanced his hidden superhuman strength.

"On one session I drank a bottle of vodka, a bottle of Thunderbird wine, two pints of Winter Warmer and then I went onto strong lager, after that six small bottles of Special Brew."

He shook his head stone-faced, incredulous now at the level of destruction he'd put his body through. These days he only drank moderately but his crack habit is a demon he can't get rid of.

"Why didn't you tell me about the hallucinations at the time, Jace?" He stared back with a confounded expression then shook his head, overwhelmed by regret.

"I'd convinced myself no-one would ever understand if I said anything. Even you, Marc. Sorry, brother. I wished I'd known what to say. How do you make someone understand something you don't understand yourself?" He considered this for a moment. "I didn't have a clue about where to begin and I was terrified of being taken away from home and sectioned or something."

I find it hard to comprehend my own inability to spot my brother's deeper problems.

"We were always close, Jason, even though you were so reclusive. You didn't speak much about anything, just sat in your room with your music on loud."

I was about to tell him how much I wished I'd understood his problems better, maybe we could all have helped. We would have certainly tried. But the past is unchangeable, we were only now at the point of understanding each other. Time spent trying to change the past is pointless, but I'll never give up on trying to make the future better for my brother.

"Look, I'd become an expert at hiding my feelings," Jason continued apologetically. "At fourteen I'd understood completely the things I saw weren't at all normal. That's why I decided to self-medicate."

Clearly, he'd quickly found himself in the grips of a Catch Twenty-Two situation. If he'd spilled the beans then, he believed, he risked being incarcerated in an institution. The facts as he considered them, as a fourteen year-old, were as clear as glass: there were quick fixes available, and everyone was doing it.

Our mother later admitted to me that she knew Jason was troubled at fourteen. But whenever she asked him if anything was the matter, a wall of denial confronted her. When he smoked a joint, he no longer looked agitated and perturbed but at ease with life. He had begun erecting his drug-fuelled force field and very quickly he'd made it impregnable.

Jason fumbled with his crack pipe, rolling it between his fingers, blowing through the mouthpiece.

"Preparing for when I leave then, Jace?" I smiled hopelessly.

"Well, I've always been honest with you, Marc. I'll never give everything up. How can I? What's the point?"

There were many points and I could have tried listing them but it was too late, his mind was set. He turned the TV on and I watched a scene play out of strange lights hovering above remote woodland where men were camping.

"I'd hate to be abducted," he muttered, unblinking.

"I'm fairly certain they'd soon drop you back on Earth, Jason."

He began thanking me for coming round and I suggested we get some food next time. His dimples erupted underneath his patchy stubble.

"I'd love that, Marc. Thanks. You're a great brother, you know that. You know I love you."

"Thanks, Jason. But you don't have to thank me so much."

He walked to the door, peeking behind the curtains through the frosted glass before opening both locks. He smirked his craggy grin and I walked out into the early summer evening, wondering what more I could really do to help my brother.

I often kick myself for never understanding fully how Jason really felt when he was fourteen, naïvely hoping he was finding the right path for his life in his own contemplative way. He was secretive and quiet. When he played music in his bedroom all day, Mum considered him just another lazy teenager. Yet he was a master of disguise, he'd slink away for a day and reappear the next, downcast and even more troubled.

I didn't know about his habit until he was nineteen and doing his Art Foundation course. As my brother always maintained, you can live a relatively normal life on smack if you look after yourself.

Perhaps if human understanding of mental illness, depression and disassociation were taught more readily at an early age we'd all have the right armament to spot the early signs. Yes, I admonish myself often, if I'd understood what course of action to take, his addictions might never have happened.

During the Seventies, Professor Bruce Alexander carried out the Rat Park Experiments. He took laboratory rats, some of which he put in solitary enclosures with no stimulation. In another enclosure he created Rat Park where there were many rats, social cohesion, toys and partners for stimulation. In each enclosure he put two water bottles, one plain, the other laced with cocaine and opiates.

In the isolation cages there was unfortunately a one hundred percent overdose rate. In Rat Park, there was almost zero percent, despite them having both bottles freely available.

The conclusion was that, if traumatised and isolated, you bond with something that provides relief and escape. The opposite of addiction isn't necessarily purely sobriety but connection, having your deepest needs met and understood by others.

12

FATHER FIGURE

It was the first day of Jason's planned heroin withdrawal, living alone in a caravan, albeit with his father as overseer. Picking him up that morning from Mum's house, I'd feared the worst but, unexpectedly, Jason was on a high. It wasn't unusual for his mood to swing chaotically between manic and ruined, so I'd braced myself, expecting to find him melancholy and depressed. After all, what did he have to look forward to for the next few weeks apart from vomiting, muscle cramps and diarrhoea? His previous attempt to withdraw using Methadone had been a stinking disaster; the stench of the chemical escaped through his skin, rivalling the resounding failure of the whole debacle.

Today, I was pleased to have my happier, whimsical brother back, if only for a brief interlude. We loaded the car, his CD collection and DVD player stuffed randomly into three flapping cardboard boxes, his selection of old coats and jackets carelessly slung into the back as if dumping them. Two black bin liners containing the rest of his clothes completed the sum of his earthly belongings. Jason covered everything with a sullied duvet, placing his favourite pillow on top like balancing the last card on top of a card stack. We were ready.

Mum looked tearfully resigned. This moment was long overdue and finally his father was going to intercede and help

Jason on the path to recovery.

"It's about time the bastard did something for him," Mum told me vehemently before we left.

My own years of resentment towards our father had passed. As a teenager, I'd suffered knowing he was living a different life with his new family. Slowly, sometimes bitterly, I adjusted to the likelihood that our father had forgotten all about us. Now the anger had been replaced by the hope that Dad would be the missing link to helping his son.

"'Bye, Mum. I'll let you know how I'm doing." Jason bent down and stroked the cat. Mum was also perplexed to see her son so chipper on such an occasion.

"Take care," she croaked, kissing him on the cheek.

Jason took off his favourite leather coat, then the sheepskin he wore underneath, revealing a worn light blue sweatshirt through which both bony elbows protruded. He flung himself into the passenger seat clutching a bulging plastic bag. As we pulled away, he showed off the contents as though they were trophies.

"The doctor's given me all the drugs I need to help me come off the gear, Marc." He looked excited. I permitted myself to laugh at the irony of how easily a large stash of drugs, albeit legal prescription highs, could fortify my brother so avidly. Paradoxically, it seemed, drugs could transform him into a confident, optimistic human as easily as they could render him a babbling, incoherent moron.

"What have you been given?" I asked out of polite curiosity. Opening the bag, he retrieved various packs and bottles, holding them out in front of him to read the name of each.

"I've got two hundred Valium…" – I swear my brother licked his lips – "…and two hundred Tramadol."

"What do they do, then?" I suddenly thought that it wouldn't be such a bad idea for me to know a bit about this mound of medicaments. Might help the toxicology report, I mused bleakly.

"They're strong painkillers. It's painful coming off gear, you know." Jason snorted a curious laugh. "And I've got two hundred

Dihydrocodeine. That's like opium." Jason sounded like a kid listing the toys he'd found in his Christmas stocking. "You get good money for these if you sell them. People do, you know? They get you pretty fucking high." He rummaged around again as I shook my head in disbelief.

"The doctor gave you all of this?"

"Yup. All of it." I struggled to believe that any doctor would equip an addict with enough fake opiates to dope the entire population of a small town. "Oh yeah. I've got two hundred Subutex as well, that helps with the symptoms of withdrawal. Cramps and joint pain. I hope I don't shit myself, Marc. You can if you're not careful."

He became quiet again then snorted his rare laugh as I considered this surreal conversation. My brother actually seemed ecstatic about his impending self-defecation and muscle spasms, not to mention the outright misery he was about to endure. I glanced at him suspiciously.

"Have you taken something, Jason?"

"I swear all I've had is a cider. Grown-ups' apple juice." He sniggered with a more familiar laugh.

"That White Star shit has never seen a fucking apple, Jason, I'll tell you that for nothing," I said.

Still, I had to be happy that he was happy and that he was committed to attempting this. He was spot on with his own assessment of his situation. After over two decades using he had to act, no-one else could do it for him. The first time he'd tried to withdraw had been a resounding failure and he began using again within forty-eight hours.

As our journey to the south coast progressed my doubts began rising, the medicines rustling inside the plastic bag troubling me. I'd heard it was dangerous for long-term dependents to come off narcotics. And I was leaving this responsibility to a man who'd not seen his son for decades and whom it was doubtful could be considered as compassionate father material. Was desperate hope making me blind? With the bag stuffed safely by his feet, Jason changed the direction of conversation.

"I saw this brilliant documentary last night," he began. "A blue whale's tongue weighs more than an elephant. It's true! And sharks can live up to a hundred years. It was an amazing programme. And do you know that, due to gravitational effects, you weigh slightly less when the moon is directly overhead? I was watching the Discovery Channel at my mate's house… they didn't really land on the moon!"

I wanted to ask what kind of documentary combined marine wildlife with lunar landings but then that was the way Jason unravelled 'facts'. Like a hamster stores food, Jason stored random facts ready to regurgitate at will and coming at you with mind-spinning velocity. It was like being beaten over the head with an encyclopaedia.

"They showed where the landing module landed. Seventeen tonnes and yet it left no impression on the surface, although the astronauts' footprints could be seen next to it. They never went to the moon, that's just what the FBI want us to believe."

"I don't do conspiracy theories," I said.

"Well, you should. They're interesting."

"Jason, did the doctor really just give you all of that medication?" There was a pause.

"Yeah." My brother's tone was as deflated as it was unconvincing.

I suspected there was another truth but I parked my inquisition, fearing I'd fuel despondency prematurely. It wasn't until a year later I learned my brother had stockpiled this medication. He'd convince the doctor on multiple occasions that he'd lost prescriptions and pilfered double supplies. Bit by bit, having hatched his plan, he'd hoarded his massive stash over a few months.

Unfortunately, his knowledge of narcotic withdrawal techniques didn't come from the doctor either but from his foolhardy clan of user associates. The other truth I discovered was that the doctor had warned him with some severity about the dangers of withdrawing alone. In fact, he'd tried to scare Jason, telling him he could be risking a brain haemorrhage or heart attack and would need constant supervision.

So much for scare tactics, Jason held his agenda. It took me a while to fully understand the real reason for his recklessness. He was about to spend time with his long-lost Dad, and nothing would be allowed to spoil that.

My own reunion with Leo, as I now thought of him, had taken place months earlier at our grandmother's funeral. Sitting in the crematorium car park I caught sight of my father arriving. Jason hadn't felt well enough to come so I endured this reunion alone, unsure about its outcome. After pensively exchanging greetings, Leo asked me how Jason was. I studied his mullet of thick grey hair and thought how the years had been kind to him. Well, he'd missed the stresses of growing up with a drug addict.

"Not good," I croaked, trying to stem my emotions. It felt weird talking with a man you knew was your father but whom you didn't recognise as such. I was nine when he left but I had little recollection as I had rarely spent any time with him. I'd learned to live without a father long before he'd left. Yet Jason always longed for his Dad.

"I'm really sorry," Leo said.

I feared for my brother's future life. Yet maybe Leo would now step in and help save his son.

Now, some months later, Jason was going to have his reunion too. From the moment he'd climbed into my car on that bright summer morning, I could tell from his expression it wasn't going to be an easy day. His pockets stuffed with tins of cider, his eyes already brimming and red. The journey along the A3 had been pensive and seemed to go on for hours as Jason twitched restlessly. At the junction for the A27, he pleaded with me to allow him to have another can.

"You promised I could have another can before we got there, Marc." It was evident from his aroma he'd already loaded himself sufficiently before leaving. "I've only had two cans, promise," he sulked miserably.

"Two cans means at least four," I snapped. I'd grown tired of listening to his familiar mantra.

"I need a drink, Marc. Please, I'm nervous."

I didn't want to appear self-righteous but I'd never understood Jason's logic that his demons could be cured by alcohol and Class As. In many ways I wanted to deliver him to our father in all his defiled beauty so Leo would get the most potent taste of his son's misery, of what my mother and I had dealt with for decades.

"Just one, Jason," I finally relented. "I want you to be a little bit sober when you finally meet him." Before I'd finished the sentence the can was half empty.

"I'm really nervous," he admitted tearfully. "What if he gives me any shit? I haven't spoken to him once since he left us." He became more irritated the more he pondered his abandonment.

"Stop winding yourself up," I commanded. "He wants to meet you. It will be what it will be."

But he was right to feel aggrieved. There had been no contact for decades. Still, it was also vital I delivered my brother only half-cut, not completely off his face. The dread of a second rejection was simultaneously the catalyst for Jason's fear and anger, and I also felt apprehensive. If our father treated Jason with anything other than kindness, the return journey would be unbearable.

Finally, from the brow of the hill on the exit road, we saw tiny white caps jumping from the tops of wavelets.

"It's a good day for a reunion, eh?"

I was trying my best. But staring nervously out of the window, Jason looked lost and bewildered, igniting a memory of him as a five year-old, staring out of the window of our father's car that last time. Four years after our move to the cottage, he'd come to collect us with a fixed agenda. Our mother silently led us to the patio while he waited on the driveway, their mutual sullenness hanging like thunderclouds. Mum waved tearfully and we watched her walk back inside the cottage. I recollect the tension between them even now with foreboding.

Our father drove in silence the short distance to a viewpoint on the Downs. We sat in silence for several minutes with Jason switching his gaze between the back of our father's head and the gliding clouds. Despite the lack of thrills, it was an outing with his Dad after all and, as we hadn't seen him in ages, Jason waited expectantly. Like a troublesome engine, it took some time for our father to get started. Finally, he stuttered into life and spoke words I remember as if it were yesterday.

"Has your mother talked to you about the exhaust?"

He glanced at us with a deadpan expression through the rearview mirror. This seemed like an absurdly serious conversation to have with our father, the most serious I ever recalled. The subject at first eluded us. Jason looked concerned, sensing that the moment at which this would all explode into happy playtime with Dad had definitely expired. He waited, mouth half-open.

"What's wrong with the exhaust?" I asked, knowing our father was the oracle on everything to do with cars and motoring.

"Not the exhaust, the divorce." Pronouncing every syllable, he shook his head slowly in the mirror. "It's when two people don't live with each other anymore."

I was nine, but I knew what the word meant. One of our friends told us he had two Dads and had used the same word. It was reassuring to know another kid understood this dynamic, especially when other kids taunted that your Dad didn't like you.

It's impossible to tell, and unfair to surmise, what our father felt about having to perform his thankless task that afternoon. It was a task demanded quite rightly by Mum, since after all it was he who'd been caught red-handed having an affair. Yet what still resonates after all these years is how dramatically Jason became undone. He sobbed bitterly, his face becoming demented as the severity of the situation sank in and we wept together.

"We're nearly there," I told Jason as we took the last turn-off. He stiffened in his seat, flicking the ring pull on another unopened can.

"No more, Jace. Please," I pleaded, as he lost all composure.

Our father's cottage was nestled in the middle of a lane with the High Street at one end and a large pond at the other. It was a quaint building, charming and alluring, the sometime traits of our father. Jason studied it with silent defiance.

My heart pounded as we walked across the bijou patio garden and readied ourselves. I reminded Jason that despite Leo being our biological father he wasn't the paternal type, hoping it would diffuse the impact of any indifference. My stomach did cartwheels again. Jason staggered slightly, steadying himself against the wall by the door. Nothing more could be done now except hope that Jason could restrain himself. He turned to me with the expression of a wounded dog, his trembling hand moving towards his coat pocket for his last unopened tin.

"No more. Wait a while longer please."

I let go of his hand and watched helplessly as he fought to contain his swirling emotions. He left the can waiting in his pocket. I knew he was pinning too much hope on a stranger but he was too vulnerable for me to tell him that at this moment. What he desired more than life was a father figure to support him, a guiding voice to help him and, most precious of all, a father who wanted his son.

My hand hovered over the knocker, quivering like a leaf. Two knocks and our father appeared hesitantly at the half-opened door.

"Aaah. How are you?" he asked, opening the door and inviting us both in. His welcome was rehearsed but convivial. Underneath this veneer he was unable to hide his shock at Jason's appearance. "Hello, Jason. How are you these days?"

He only had to look. With a flash of sad rage, it struck me how old Jason looked in comparison. The juxtaposition of our well-groomed father in his crisp white shirt and faded jeans, still giving the appearance of a hipster in his dotage, and my addled brother coming apart, was poignant.

He put his hand out stiffly and the two men shook hands, Jason swaying like a twig in a breeze, inebriated, eyes brimming. Their similarity struck me like a hammer blow. Leo was the older, shorter version of Jason, whose gangly frame dwarfed him. Our father's vigorous silver mullet mirrored Jason's, which was just propagating the seeds of greyness.

"Come on inside." Leo beckoned to us but Jason became more hesitant.

"I'll have a cigarette here first." He produced his pouch of Golden Virginia and our father did the same. Although it was late February, the front patio was a suntrap with enough warmth to sit outside comfortably. With a mild grunt, Leo limped to the furthest chair. As if petitioning for pity, he informed us that his hip was playing up. He was an older man now in his mid-seventies, even though he didn't look it. We sat around a circular iron table as they rolled their cigarettes in awkward silence, formulating words in their minds. With his chin slumped on his chest, Jason admired his cigarette with avid concentration as a succession of tears trickled down his cheeks.

"Marc has told me you've had a few problems over the years." It was meant to be a careful probe.

"A few?" my brother snorted incredulously. "I'm a fucking drug addict." Jason cuffed his tears and stared at his father defiantly.

On the outside I tried appearing calm and collected. Inside, my intestines were churning. This was going to go one of two ways. Their interaction was justifiably awkward. Watching my father's gaze stray between my brother and myself, I earnestly needed him to help my brother. If he could do that one thing, I could pardon his previous neglect.

I've always had empathy for Jason, but this was another first as it was the first compassion I've ever felt for my father. It was an awful reality to confront, even for a man who was never much of a Dad. He was fumbling for something more to say.

"He's very nervous," I interceded. "He's had a few cans on the way down, as you can see." My brother needed someone to represent his case better than himself. He wasn't always this way after all. The two men blew smoke above their heads, before Jason sat himself upright and looked directly at Leo.

"What do you want us to call you? I'm not calling you Dad."

Our father looked flummoxed. "I'll call you Leo if you don't mind," said my brother, looking at him angrily.

"Jason, come on. Let's keep it civil," I appealed.

It was evident that in his solitary meditations over the years, Jason had rehearsed many things he wanted to say to his father. Whilst I'd moved on from the hurt, Jason still languished in the past. He was entitled to say whatever he wanted to his father but I feared he'd jeopardise any ongoing relationship if he wasn't reigned in a bit. I needed another ally. And Dads are supposed to help their kids when they need them.

"Are you with anyone at the moment?" our father asked, as I reminded myself to breathe.

"I've got a girlfriend called Diane." For a moment it seemed likely a civil conversation would ensue. "She's an alcoholic." Jason puffed his smoke across the table.

"You seem a little upset, Jason," said Leo, and my anxiety started round two.

"It's been a tough few weeks," my brother muttered miserably, as the tears gained momentum. "My friend Davey took an overdose a few weeks ago and died." Jason then reeled off a list of dead people he'd once known before his chin slumped on his chest again. "Look, I'm sorry but I'm an addict. I just need a fix," he announced. "That's the way it is."

He got to his feet clutching a small plastic bag, looking first at our father and then me.

"I need to use your toilet for a moment, to sort myself out," he added, as if it wasn't clear what he needed to do.

13

THE CARAVAN TRIALS

L eo looked completely out of his depth as we sat out on the patio. He hadn't envisaged this scenario. How could I have prepared him for the likelihood that his youngest son might need to inject heroin during their reunion? When I'd told him at the funeral that Jason was 'not good' I wasn't kidding. Leo tried to say something but words failed him. What could he say? By drinking heavily, Jason had tried to stave off the inevitable; but now at this moment of despair, there was nothing more he could do and a hit was the only remedy.

"Where's the bathroom?" my brother demanded. Leo gave directions and Jason disappeared inside.

"It's just hopeless, isn't it?" Leo said. Raising his eyebrows, he emitted a hollow laugh. "Everyone's an alcoholic or drug addict or dead by the looks of things." His sour humour provoked a shallow smile of resignation from me.

"I told you things weren't good."

"Is he always like this?"

I felt a shimmer of rage. He'd never had to deal with the problems and drudgery Jason's life presented and now he was already frustrated.

"He has better days," I reassured him. "This is hard for him emotionally." As he sighed with exasperation I felt my resentment escalate. This reunion was proving trickier than I'd envisaged. "It must be hard dealing with a drug addict son needing to take a hit in your toilet." Trying to be magnanimous gave me the resolve to endure the awkwardness.

"Well, it's all so hopeless for him, isn't it? What's to be done?" Our father watched his cigarette smoke curl up silently as two swans padded past the gate. "They're buggers, those swans." The birds waddled past like two old men.

"Why's that?"

"They go up to the end of the street to the corner shop and nick fruit from the display, then waddle back to the pond. Sometimes Amrit gives chase. It's like a Python sketch." My father cracked with infectious laughter and for ten minutes we were a father and son, enjoying a moment of uncomplicated togetherness. Then Jason reappeared, the bag containing his works wrapped tightly in his hand.

"Sorry, I'm ill. I can't help it." He looked at us remorsefully, his face now serene. My brother was now normal again, sensitive and thoughtful. "That's the trouble with the brown," he explained, shaking his head dismayed. "Those first few hits mean you spend the rest of your life struggling to stay healthy and needing more and more of the stuff. I'd tell anyone who wanted to try it not to waste their time. It's a waste of money…" – he thought some more – "…a waste of fucking life," he snorted.

Our father then asked his son the golden question.

"What do you want to do, Jason? You can't spend the rest of your life like this can you?" Yes! I was jubilant. This is what I'd hoped, that Dad would intervene and become the catalyst for a dramatic change in Jason's fortunes. "What do you want to do with your life?" he repeated, and Jason mulled the question over amidst a haze of cigarette smoke.

"I want to get off the gear. I've got to or I've got no chance."

I waited for him to protest, as he'd done before, about how you could expect a normal lifespan and still take heroin if you took care of yourself and didn't take too much. But that was a futile argument. What quality of life would that be? And anyhow, my brother never could control his intake. The drugs he needed to stop his torment controlled him.

"I need to get away from the dealers where I live. And other users. I need to go somewhere and come off the gear."

"Well. We'll have to get our heads together, then, won't we?" Leo replied.

Jason made another visit on his own after this reunion and had a breakthrough in his relationship with his father.

Leo's promise to reimburse Jason's train fare meant everything to him. He could be confident that his father actually wanted to see him, not just because his conscience was nagging him. Jason didn't hide behind his addictions this time; he was straight and full of stories to tell his Dad. Leo even took him to his local for lunch and introduced him as his son to his drinking pals. When Jason joyfully told me about this excursion, I began feeling the shoots of fondness for the stranger that was our father. For him, in turn, their meeting proved that his youngest was really trying to better his life and wanted support, not cash.

"It was awkward at first," Jason reported to me later. Our father had been painting a wooden fence in the garden when he arrived. "He was painting like he'd never held a brush in his life. I know he can fake a Rembrandt, but he can't paint a fucking fence." Jason laughed as he told the story. He'd watched patiently, before realising that at his father's pace there'd be no drinking time left. "I snatched the brush from his hand and said let me do it. It'll be much quicker."

I laughed, remembering the last time he'd done some painting for me. 'Quicker' didn't equate to tidy efficiency, as I recalled the thick splatters of colour on the doorstep and the windowpanes.

"He jumped when I snatched the brush and I asked him if he

was scared of me," Jason told me.

"Yes. A bit," Leo admitted.

"Well, do be," Jason had said uncharacteristically.

He was never an aggressive person. However, his residual anger at his father's past indifference clearly still lingered. Apparently, Leo resigned himself to watching Jason paint the remainder of the fence in under an hour, leaving plenty of time for the pub.

My father was a well-known face at his local. The two of them wandering into The Blue Bell like a couple of Rolling Stones must have been an intriguing sight. He introduced his lost son to his friends and it had been a resounding success, according to Jason.

"They all liked me in there," he said triumphantly. As they'd left the pub and taken the short route across the car park, Leo had stopped abruptly.

"I'm proud of you," he told Jason. I could hardly see through my own welling tears as my brother reported this.

"What have you got to be proud of?" Jason asked, always honest and self-deprecating.

"The way you got on so well with everyone and the way you conducted yourself in there."

"He didn't mention your fence painting skills, then, Jason?" I had to quip.

As I drove us south again for his next visit, Jason looked happy. Something was healing. He told me that before leaving he'd asked Leo if he could now call him Dad and our father had simply replied, "Yes."

The clear span of turquoise water came into view at the final junction and I felt cautiously happy. The honeymoon was now going to be celebrated in a pool of sickness and diarrhoea, the venue a shabby metal shed on wheels that our father had sourced for the purpose, situated a few convenient miles from where he lived.

When we arrived at the cottage this time, the atmosphere was convivial and easy. The familiarity with which Jason interacted with his father astonished me at first and I felt like the outsider.

But as I watched Jason breeze around the kitchen I could tell from Leo's expression that he shared my concern about how this withdrawal would pan out. My brother looked at us both and smiled, the lines around his eyes creasing like starbursts as he contentedly snapped the ring pull on another can.

"Can't give up everything at once." He cocked the can at us with a wink.

Jason was feeling well at this point. We ate a lunch our stepmother had prepared that morning, balancing the plates on our laps in the small living room. With the meal finished, seeing no reason to prolong the inevitable, we decided it was time to get Jason settled in. A flutter of concern twisted a knot in my stomach. My brother's suffering would soon begin.

It was an easy route along a single snaking country road to the caravan site, one intended for residents not holidaymakers. It was tidy, populated by an eclectic mix of caravans of assorted sizes and older ones rescued from other sites. Having parked up we grabbed some of Jason's belongings and followed Leo through the maze of homes. Most were large two- and three-bed static caravans, flower boxes populating windowsills or surrounding wooden decking.

Not too shabby, I thought, before spotting the caravan we were approaching. The key Leo produced to unlock it resembled the one I have for my garden shed. We walked straight into a tiny lounge where a decrepit TV sat on a small table in the corner.

"The owner of the site said you could keep that," our father informed Jason.

A little natural light entered the room through the dirty nets at the double window and the blue-grey carpet tiles were worn and in need of an upgrade. But the caravan smelled like it had been freshly cleaned. Leo and his wife had put some time and effort into making it habitable. I remembered a room I'd once rescued Jason from in the truly bad times. I left his dirty mattress on the filthy floorboards upon discovering the dirty syringes that he and the other inhabitants had stashed underneath. This caravan was a palace in comparison.

"You've got no rent to worry about for a few months," our father declared proudly. "And I've got these for you." He showed Jason the small second-hand electric cooker in the kitchen. "The fridge is brand new." In a small room next to the kitchen was a toilet and shower. He opened the door like an estate agent and pointed to the toiletries. "You've got some new shower gel and soap."

"That's great, thanks. Where's the bedroom?" Jason was an eager beaver that afternoon, his forehead already beginning to bead with perspiration. Leo marched us from the kitchen, through the lounge to the back of the caravan. The double bed was furnished with clean bedclothes. Jason surveyed the room with contentment and patted the mattress. "I'll be spending a lot of time in here for the next few weeks." He laughed, contemplating this prospect contentedly.

"I'll get the rest of your stuff, Jason."

I left them. I didn't rush. I wanted my brother to discuss things with his father about ongoing care. There had already been talk of him registering with a local doctor. I relinquished the reins of responsibility uneasily. I could hardly blame Leo for having no clue about how much support Jason would need since his track record on parental care was non-existent.

In the lounge we amassed Jason's artefacts and belongings and I suggested I give our father a lift back so Jason could organise himself for a while before I returned. The two men shared another friendly handshake and my father invited Jason to come down later to see him for some dinner. As we left, I detected the creeping signs of trepidation in Jason. He looked vulnerable as he surveyed his belongings in the middle of the lounge like a puzzle.

"I'll be back in a while, Jason," I reassured him.

I returned with a handful of good luck cards I'd collected from family members. Inside, I discovered the duvet, pillow and DVD player had been taken to the bedroom and ceremoniously dumped in an untidy pile on the bed, the electric cable wrapped around the pillow.

"It's a nice place, isn't it?" Jason said, wiping his brow. He appeared content but it saddened me seeing how easily pleased he could become. He was waiting for my endorsement.

"It's better than that shithole you were in before," I agreed.

I thought back to when I'd collected Jason earlier. He'd called to warn me that the man he was subletting from would use a Stanley knife on me if I came into the building. To my surprise, though, his tormentor leapt out of the kitchen window when I banged hard on the door and shouted my brother's name loudly, a hammer tucked into my belt. I felt confident that at least this was a safer environment and he had his father to look after him.

Jason cooed over the five cards I handed him, touched and humbly surprised by the support he had behind him. This solidarity meant everything to him. He moved a small armchair aside. On the right was an electric fire with a narrow mantelpiece above.

"There will be good," he said, meticulously placing each card on the mantelpiece, smiling at them. "Thanks, Marc, for everything you do for me. Thanks. You're a good brother. You know I love you."

I made coffee and brought one through for him, black and strong the way he always liked it. He was attempting in vain to get reception on the TV, which hissed white noise in defiance. When he opened the window and hung the aerial outside, indiscernible shapes began moving on the screen.

"You can't leave the aerial hanging out." I thought about rain and wind and the neighbours.

"I'll sort it later when you've gone," he said, looking increasingly unsettled. "I need things to do." I watched the growing bead of perspiration on his upper lip. As we drank coffee, I ran through the list of food we'd bought, making sure he had everything he needed.

"Don't worry," he mustered a smile. "I've got these to help me." He shook the blue plastic bag. "And these." He reached inside his coat to retrieve further cans of White Star he'd stashed away, placing them alongside the cards on the mantelpiece. "The doctor said I can't give up the booze as well. It's too dangerous."

Jason was starting his first day of withdrawal with a curious concoction, enough prescription opiates to decimate the caravan park along with copious chemical cider to wash away the taste.

"Sure you'll be okay? Call me if you need anything." I was hesitant about leaving.

"I'll be fine. I know I've just got to do this, Marc. Dad says he'll look after me." Jason suddenly looked content as he wiped the sweat from his face. Perhaps Dad was all he really needed.

Leaving Jason wasn't easy. I chuckled, though, closing the door and hearing him furiously thumping the top of the TV while still thanking me profusely for everything I'd done.

"And thank everyone for the cards, Marc."

I walked to my car and wept for five hard minutes.

The days of torture commenced as expected. Jason's torment gained momentum shortly after I'd left. According to the medical people, the worst reactions usually peak in a few days but can linger for several weeks. Jason's experience superseded this prognosis.

He told me that the first three weeks without sleep were the worst. We'll never know how credible his claim was. What an addict often terms as the 'love affair', the craving for the substance that enables their being, lasts for months, sometimes years, perhaps a lifetime. This would be his ongoing battle.

With his pill and booze concoction, he supplemented his withdrawal with a rich cacophony of music, his life's soundtrack. As his mind grew restless he rode the muscle spasms and unfathomable despondency with his tunes. When the cramps and pain grew strong and dark, he blasted Black Sabbath or Led Zeppelin loudly from his CD player, the tinny speakers crackling in distress. When the cramps subsided, he passed the brief tranquility with Neil Young, sometimes a touch of Crosby Stills & Nash, music in synchronicity with despair. Although the sounds helped the anguish, they also mostly eased his loneliness as he recalled good memories of the parties, the drugs and the happy mayhem he'd enjoyed.

The side effects of withdrawal and misery he'd fully expected, and I'll always admire his fortitude to endure in the face of such adversity unaccompanied. Yet Jason informed me, when I revisited a week later, that his despair had unexpectedly attracted another visitor during the first night he spent alone in the caravan.

He'd gone to bed at midnight after another bitter feud with the TV set, despairing of ever seeing anything on it. Having tried a couple more tins of White Star, some Tramadol and a couple of Valium, he wasn't quite yet in need of the Dihydrocodeine. Instead, having digested some information about red wine's powerful antioxidant qualities, he decided to retire with a bottle. The tremors and spasms were getting worse and the caravan's toilet system had already been well and truly tested.

With the duvet wrapped around him, he'd begun sweating profusely. But removing himself from his cocoon, he quickly became cold again, and the cycle of fluctuating temperature became a steady rhythm. After enduring this torment for several hours, he returned to the lounge where he sat in the armchair in despair. Surveying the room he noticed the horizontal bars of the electric heater glowing hot and red and the five good luck cards he'd meticulously placed on the mantle were in the order he'd originally left them... but upside down.

"It follows me, Marc," he cried. "Always. It's even followed me down here."

As far as I could comprehend, 'it' had a name, it was mental illness and it was Jason's despairing mind suffering the comedown of narcotic withdrawal. But my brother was insistent that 'it' was more insidious than a mental disturbance. It had a personality that had warped from the days he conversed with it reticently in his bedroom as a child, onto the present when it tormented him by knocking on his wall or calling out his name at night.

"And I didn't put the fire on, I promise," he insisted. "I turned it off at the wall as well and pulled out the plug."

Why Jason took these precautions, if true, intrigued me. Next, he said, he turned off the heater and replaced the cards then went back to his bedroom and climbed under the duvet. The Tramadol was taking effect and the Valium was easing his anxiety. He felt satisfied and safe within his veil, nothing could touch him; he took two more Valium, he was again invincible. He lived by the motto that nothing could torture his soul more than the torture he'd already endured. If all else failed, he had antioxidant red wine to fortify himself and purge his system of the poison.

But the spiral of hot and cold sweats, spasms and fever continued until he couldn't bear it any longer. He returned to the lounge where again he discovered the heater angry and red, the cards now face down on the carpet and scattered across the floor.

As I write of the despair my brother later chronicled, I feel remorse that I couldn't have been there to help. He'd been insistent that the first few days he wanted to be able to puke, shit and despair in private. He had Dad looking out for him anyway, didn't he?

For the first two weeks there was a strict routine. At lunchtime, our father picked him up, took him back to his cottage and give him food. An hour later he'd drop him back to the caravan where Jason endured another night's torment. I'm sure Leo found himself out of his depth quite quickly. Staying with his son longer than an hour was unbearable but at least he'd tried. Typically, Jason, sensitive to his father's perception and not wanting to be perceived as a complete head case, kept the worst of his torments to himself, only sharing them when I called or came to visit.

Jason didn't know his neighbours and they didn't know him. He was alone except for phone calls from a few concerned family members. Diane, his girlfriend, informed him one night that she'd entered a rehabilitation centre for alcohol dependency having been told a few more drinks would finally plunder her frail body.

Along with the knowledge that he finally held his father's attention, this gave my brother solace, knowing that by his own actions he was miraculously empowering others to follow.

14

I'M NOT MAD

"**B**efore you arrived, I was thinking about that flat me and Diane had," said Jason. He tried to light a cigarette, flicking his hair back over his ear and away from the roaring flame of the Zippo, puffing frantically. The evidence of years of neglect, the dark bruised patches populating his sinewy arms, were highlighted by the flickering flame. The scene was reminiscent of a bleak Russian novel. I readied myself for another story that, he believed, conclusively proved the supernatural intervention he'd experienced all his life to be true. This time it had a witness.

As they sat on their mattress in the filthy south London flat, Jason and Diane had noticed a slowly pulsing light seeping from under the door of the bedroom. Jason rolled a cigarette, trying to work out what he was actually seeing while Diane reached for a wiry brown blanket and snuggled her frail body under it. She observed Jason as he littered the mattress with flecks of tobacco. They both stared at the palpitating light passing under the door.

They shared the flat with other dysfunctional tenants but it was late and they felt sure the others had long since gone to bed. The house was silent. And despite living chaotic lives, my brother and his girlfriend always meticulously checked the communal lights were switched off each night before they went to bed.

Jason flicked his lighter on, holding the flame towards Diane's face to check she was awake and sharing the same vision, another misplaced flashback perhaps? At the corner of the mattress, her dark eyes stared intently at the oscillating light in the gap beneath the door.

"Did you switch the light off, Jace?" she asked, her eyes still fixated. "You didn't leave the oven on or anything?" For a moment, Diane considered whether the weird pulsating light could be the result of a fire that had started in the communal kitchen.

"No! I turned the fucking lights off and I haven't used the cooker for days," Jason insisted, his eyes glued to the light infiltration. "It's not a fire either," Jason rationalised. "There's no smoke."

"Go and see what it is, Jace," Diane pleaded, giving him a timid push with her trembling hand. "I don't like it. It's weird."

Standing in his night attire, dirty torn thermals and squalid tee-shirt, Jason moved warily towards the light, finding and gulping down a half-empty tin of White Star on the way. Reaching the handle of the door, uneasiness swept through him. Unsure of what he'd find beyond, he was nevertheless aware these happenings weren't unusual in his life. He pulled the door open slowly.

"What is it?" Desperate and uneasy, Diane just wanted to sleep.

In the silence of the landing, Jason listened to his own heavy breathing. The light was coming from the kitchen to his right. Watching its pulsation and rhythm, he felt relieved, perhaps Diane was right and it was a fire. With this strangely comforting rationale he pushed open the kitchen door... and stared in disbelief at the glowing orbs of light hovering above the kitchen table. Orange, red and swirling, they began billowing around him.

"It was like being in some psychedelic bubble factory," he told me.

He described how the largest 'mother orb' pulsated above the table, surrounded by many smaller orbs, pulsating faster. Their undulations and changes of size and colour became more enigmatic the further he ventured into the room, making him believe they were aware of him. As the mother orb expanded and contracted, he felt he was being examined in some unexplainable way.

Jason stared back in astonishment and their dance momentarily stopped as he ventured closer to the table, within touching distance. An air of inquisitiveness seemed to ripple through them as they rose and fell, like apples bobbing in an unseen astral river.

Behind him, he heard the floorboards creak and turned to stare at Diane, waif-like, standing just shy of the kitchen entrance, the blanket draped around her shoulders. In their shared moment, the whole world outside ceased to exist. Jason beckoned Diane inside and she stood beside him as they watched the dancing orbs in silent disbelief. Turning to face each other, Jason said he watched their reflection dancing within her incredulous brown eyes. Then one by one they began to disappear.

"You see, Marc, Diane saw the orbs too. She watched with me."

It was true. Diane had told our mother the same crazy story a day later. I considered it one of the inexplicable reasons they'd maintained their closeness. With Diane, my brother believed he'd found a soulmate, he was no longer a loner who experienced strange manifestations. As he sparked another cigarette, I remembered his stories of the orbs outside his bedroom window at Fir Tree Cottage. This latest experience was not his alone but irrefutable proof that it was a reality.

"So what did you do once the orbs disappeared?" I asked him. I treated Jason's claims agnostically but with consideration, curious how anyone could move on from an experience like this, imagined or otherwise.

He explained that the mother orb was the last to extinguish. Then they had crept back to their bedroom where, holding hands, they resumed their positions slumped against the wall. In the darkness Jason put his mouth gently to Diane's ear.

"I told you I saw these things. I told you," he whispered.

But that wasn't the end of the story.

A few days later, Jason had entered the flat late one afternoon frantic for a fix. He went to retrieve his works from his hiding place under the bedroom floorboards. No-one knew about this hiding place, not even Diane. Reaching his hand deep under the floorboards, he padded around the void trying to locate his stash, the cling-filmed parcel he'd placed between two joists and covered with a stained tea towel. Cursing and sweating, the need for a fix possessed him. But, to his dismay, the stash was nowhere.

Despairing, he began pulling up the floorboards, some splintering as he ripped them up. The evidence was overwhelming as he glared into the empty void: his stash was gone. He succumbed to total paranoia. Weeping with misery, he concluded that someone had stolen it. There were six people sharing the house and one was Diane.

She returned to a frantic inquisition. Jason assaulted her with questions, his tone uncharacteristically hostile, leaving her shocked and bewildered. Over and over he asked if she or any of the other scum they shared the flat with knew of his hiding place. Growing progressively distressed, he'd fled, desperate to find a backup fix.

Returning to their bedroom in the early evening, Jason realised his surroundings were not as he'd left them. To his astonishment, his works were not only back but had been deliberately arranged on the floor in front of him. The cling-filmed bag, dirty dishcloth, burnt silver foil and box of Swan Vesta had been arranged in a meticulous line across the floorboards, punctuated with two used syringes. The assembly, Jason said examining it closely, resembled some kind of mathematical equation. The scene perplexed him.

"Sorry I was horrible to you, Di," he whispered later that night as they lay on their mattress. He kissed her and, once she was asleep, bundled the remnants of the stash and hid them away again.

"You hid them in the same place?" I asked.

"Yes. Back where no-one could find them." Jason stared at me innocently. "It wasn't Diane or anyone else. It was whatever follows me."

A couple of years later, Jason stared at his phone ringing on the kitchen worktop. The contact name 'Mum' lit brightly on the screen sobered him. He didn't know why he had a sinking feeling so he hesitated, his hand hovering above the shabby mobile. But he couldn't ignore it.

"Hello."

"Where are you, Jason?"

"I'm round Gavin's house. Why?" he asked, suspicious of her tone. He fixed a shameful gaze on the yellowed glass pipe resting against an open tube of bicarbonate of soda on the worktop. Like finding himself unexpectedly naked, Jason felt guilty about his afternoon's indulgencies.

"Can you come back home, Jason? I need to talk to you." He looked across at Gavin slumped in an armchair in the corner of his cramped living room, staring mindlessly at the TV.

"When do you want me back?" He hoped it was just trivia keeping him from another toke of the tiny white rock nestled in the top of his pipe.

"Pop over now, please." Sensing his apprehension, she reassured him convivially, "You're not in trouble or anything. I just need to talk to you in person."

"Okay, I'll be two minutes," he replied. Slipping on his dishevelled leather overcoat, he smiled at Gavin. "Gotta go back to Mum's for a bit. See yer later, yeah?"

"Seeya, Neo," Gav whispered catatonically.

Jason left, unable to shift his sense of unease, pulling his overcoat close to shield himself from the wind funnelling through the ally. Despite the guilt he felt about his afternoon's indulgencies, he reminded himself he'd actually been quite good in comparison to the old days. There was a time, he remembered with fondness, when he wouldn't have been able to resist a last little crack crystal or a smattering of brown still left on a burnt scrap of tin foil.

With every step, he thought about all the efforts he'd made in life to fight his addiction urges. He felt proud about weaning himself off heroin, alone in that shitty caravan. On the other hand, he knew he was seamlessly slipping into old habits. The brown he once relied on had changed to white. His meditative steps continued until he acknowledged dismally that, in reality, not much in his life had changed at all despite his struggles.

The natural high he'd gained from kicking heroin had been short-lived once he returned home from his ten-month stint on the south coast. Having done the hardest thing he'd ever done, he felt a fool for believing life would suddenly open its arms with opportunities.

Approaching Mum's house, Jason braced himself for an inquisition. He could never understand how she could tell he'd been using when he felt confident he could conceal the effects so well. He could handle drugs and alcohol better than anyone else he knew. Could she smell it on his clothes? What was it she detected anyway? A vagueness in his eyes? An unsteadiness? These questions possessed him anxiously as he pressed the doorbell.

"How are you, Jason?" Mum looked down on her son standing below on the bottom doorstep like a windswept scarecrow. Jason tried smiling as she observed him with a look of concern he didn't understand. Why hadn't her drug detection radar gone off yet? She gestured for him to come in from the cold and he stepped through the door in baffled silence. "Do you want a coffee? Have you eaten anything today?"

"I'll have a coffee, Mother. Thank you. Black, yeah?" He followed her into the kitchen nervously.

"Jason, I think I can remember how you have your coffee." She mustered a smile whilst inwardly gripped by fear of how he'd receive the news she was about to give him. "What have you been up to today, anyway?" She already knew the answer, of course, she could see it in his eyes, smell it on his clothes. For once she felt glad he'd numbed himself.

"So, what do you want to talk to me about? If it's about my bedroom, I'll clean it later, I promise." Jason tried ignoring another pang of unease about the drug paraphernalia poorly hidden among the garbage tip of his old bedroom. Shaking her head, Mum took a gulp of coffee, bracing herself for the awful inevitable.

"I'm afraid Diane died today, Jason," she said, fighting back emotions.

Mum was fond of Diane, as were we all. Sometimes she felt the same level of empathy for her as for her own son, alongside despair at Diane's dysfunctional ways, angry that she too was incapable of helping herself. Jason gripped the worktop, staring hard at his mother, his mouth agape, his eyes already laden with tears.

"What happened to her?" he asked incredulously.

"Sit down, Jason." With her hand on his arm she coaxed him towards a chair at the table, apprehensive about his instability, both physical and mental.

"I knew she'd come out of rehab six months ago," he said. "They put her in a dry house."

"I think she was thrown out for having a relationship with a fellow inmate," Mum said. Jason wiped the tears from his eyes and misery from his nose. He already knew about Diane's previous dalliance. "I'm sorry to tell you, really. Peter told us this morning and I needed to tell you before you heard it elsewhere."

"He probably blames me. I wasn't with her though. She was with that new bloke. He was a total pisshead as well."

"How did you know about her new boyfriend, Jason?"

"I've been talking to her on the phone a lot recently." Jason's voice cracked, remembering her fragility and kind, gentle smile. He recalled her laugh, the way it wriggled through her entire body. They were infectious traits that he'd loved about her. "She'd been asking about me through people we knew. So I gave her a call a few months back."

"I'm sorry, Jason. It must be hard, you were with her for a long time."

"Thirteen years, on and off. I was with her when they assessed her for rehab. That was nearly two years ago. Then they detected alcohol on her when she first went to live at the Centre and refused her entry." Mum watched Jason's tears stop as he now became angry. "I asked to see the manager of the place."

"Jason, why would they listen to you? You're an addict as well." Mum didn't want to debate semantics but his claims were sometimes too unbearable to leave unchallenged.

"Straight up, I promise. They let me go in and talk to the manager and I told him, you have to take her in or she'll die."

"And they agreed with you?" Mum asked, surprised.

"Yes. It was me that got her into rehab. They agreed to try and save her, she'd have died otherwise. They'd have thrown her out before she'd even started." Jason recalled the conversation he'd had at the Centre. "They told me they'd never made an allowance before when someone was positive with alcohol."

There was a close bond between Jason and Diane. She'd been a source of inspiration while he endured the cramps and misery of his own withdrawal. Her attempts to get clean from acute alcohol dependency had kept him motivated.

"I remember her phoning me from rehab when I was in that caravan coming off the gear." Jason's tears flowed as he described how Diane's calls helped him in his darkest moments, with the loneliness of a shed on wheels in a place he didn't know, plagued by an unseen tormentor. "I used to come up and see her every few months once I was clean and well enough."

"She was lucky she had you then, Jason. You should be pleased you helped her as well. At least she got some extra life." Mum embraced his account, knowing how Jason always tries to do his best. He's a caring and loving person.

"I suppose." Staring at the ceiling, Jason searched for other silver linings. "Do you remember the state she was in before going into rehab?" Mum nodded silently. "She spent six weeks in ICU before she got the rehab place. The hospital gave her an ultimatum, stop drinking or die. I know I'm no role model, but I did try to help her stop when I was with her." Jason blew his nose before saying bitterly, "Maybe if she hadn't been with me she would've got sober sooner."

The years of drinking had left Diane with acute cirrhosis and her health hanging by a thread when she entered the dry house. But after succumbing to old habits, she inevitably lost her life.

Mum watched his tears cascade again, racking her mind for an anecdote she could ease his regrets with. If she couldn't, she knew he'd find other ways to escape the pain upstairs in his bedroom later.

"Do you think she wanted to get back with you, Jason?" she tried.

"It looked that way. I went and saw her and she told me she missed me and wanted to finish with her new bloke."

He paused, trying to regain composure. There would be no future relationship with Diane now. The sad hypothesis I believe is that, despite her love for Jason, Diane knew he wasn't the best person to be with and she fought against her love for him like another addiction. They were no match made in Heaven. But for Jason, if he thought about whether Heaven even existed, Diane would have been the one sharing it with him.

Along with my brother's regrets over this relationship, I had one of my own, a regret that had nagged me from a year before her spell in rehab. Late one afternoon, between the cars streaming down the main road, I'd noticed a forlorn woman on the other side of the road. It wasn't recognition that initially caught my eye but her abject sadness. Scrunched on a wooden bench, her skinny arms wrapped around her legs and chin resting on top of her knees, she stared vacantly at the YMCA opposite, a cigarette resting between her fingers.

Commuters filed past, hindering my view, but clearly the years had been cruel and she possessed a haunting vulnerability. Struggling to relight her cigarette with a shaking hand, she leaned in and puffed fervently, releasing a plume of grey-blue smoke. I remained motionless as she continued staring blankly through the smoky haze. Standing on the edge of the curb I waited for an oncoming bus to pass.

I'd not seen Diane for years and I felt a duty to her to make sure she was okay, to see if she needed anything. She'd been a good friend in what seemed like another lifetime. Her children had grown up with my own. Finally, the bus passed and I crossed to find the bench empty. I glanced around and caught a glimpse of her vanishing inside the YMCA, the last time I saw her despite looking for her every time I passed.

Jason cried with Mum until the early hours. Diane's death traumatised him more than he could comprehend and he was loaded with sorrow and regret.

"I've never been part of this world," he wailed, fists clenched, angry at life's challenges and hardships that he could only control with drugs.

"You have to get clean, Jason, once and for all. You can't keep on like this." Jason looked at our mother through bitter tears, knowing she spoke the truth. Somehow, like me, she always held onto a little piece of hope.

"My life's a fucking nightmare," he said.

"It will get better once you're straight. But you can't substitute one addiction with another. You have to be clean of everything."

Later, Jason would tell me what happened next and clearly still barely believed it himself.

Exhausted, he'd gone up to his bedroom. Climbing into bed, a wave of calmness filled him and he remembered slipping to sleep immediately. Then in the early hours he woke, aware of something disturbing him. Lifting his head, he searched the room for abnormality, his usual routine. Lying on the mattress he sensed swaying movement. He hadn't drunk enough to induce the woozy sensation he was experiencing, the small lampshade above him growing and reducing in size as he stared at it. He wondered if his eyes were just playing tricks.

Anxiety pricked him alert. Sitting upright gave him a better view of the door of the tiny bedroom, its horizontal and vertical panels moving from side to side, up and down. Jason realised then his bed was jumping around uncontrollably, the energy and force strong and unstoppable. With a thump, the wooden legs of the bed pounded rhythmically onto the floor with a drumming tremor.

Jason's terror and bewilderment was evident as he relived the episode. Was he dreaming or hallucinating? Composing himself from the shock, the bed rose and swayed like a bucking bronco before doing a further aggressive shake.

Through a gap in the curtains he tried focusing on the sky outside. Was it still night-time? Was it getting lighter? Believing he was awake and that nothing he could do would stop the horror, he mustered a cry to Mum. His words rose but no sound came out. He tried again in desperation, this time his cry louder and he heard it resonate. With a shuddering bump and a few last defiant gyrations the bed stilled. The room became silent. The curtain shifted as a gentle breeze meandered through the room. Climbing to his feet, Jason scrabbled at the door and from the corner of his eye noticed the bed faintly shudder again.

Outside his door he gazed across at Mum's bedroom opposite listening to his racing heartbeat punching angrily at his chest. The fear overpowered him and only one thing could pacify him. He looked longingly at the dull light seeping under Mum's door. Suddenly it flew open. Flicking on the landing light she stood staring at him, bewildered.

"Jason! What are you doing? What was all that noise?"

"My fucking bed was jumping around the room!" he declared, like a child appealing to a disapproving parent.

My brother gazed at me accusingly as he told this story. I felt

167

terrible for my sudden befuddled laughter as I pictured the frown on our mother's face at his absurd reply.

"What have you taken, Jason?" Understandably, she'd concluded he was high again, feeling foolish for believing things would ever change. He protested tearfully that he hadn't touched a thing, frustrated by the accusation while his fear still felt so raw and powerful. "Go back to bed. It's three in the morning," she said, her tone softening.

Although exasperated, it must have destroyed her to see her son hopelessly in the depths of despair. She admitted to me later that she often pleaded to a higher being for an answer as to how best to help him. She never got an answer.

Jason stumbled downstairs disconsolately, sliding his hand along the banister. Collecting his dirty coat in the hallway he made his way into the living room, lay on the couch and once again thought about his father. He had always loved his father.

15

TROUBLED

Standing at the top of the short steps to his new home, Jason looked pleased as punch. It was a tiny terrace house, the kitchen leading left from the sitting room, a single bedroom and miniscule bathroom upstairs.

"The council finally came through for me. It's nice. It's a cracking place," he smiled in disbelief. Suddenly he shot past me into his kitchen, shouting over his shoulder. "Thanks for everything you do for me, Marc. You're such a good brother. I do appreciate it. You're a great brother. Thank you for everything you do for me."

As usual, my hand went up to silence him. He always overdid his praise. That's what brothers are meant to do for each other, isn't it? Even if that help needs to last a lifetime.

I felt that at last we were getting somewhere with him. There was a discernible light at the end of the tunnel. It was good to be pleased about his progress, it had taken many years to feel this way. Was his manic helter-skelter ride really coming to rest? I hoped so. It had been draining. Jason was keeping his appointments with the mental health team and, more importantly, he was doing things for himself. I considered him as someone with prospects.

I looked around for somewhere to sit. There were two black plastic chairs in his sitting room which a friend had loaned to him. I reminded him I'd be dropping my old two-seater sofa round later along with a comfortable armchair he could watch TV from. His friends were all couch-hoppers anyway so I knew they'd come in handy.

Generally his 'friends' conducted any transactions for gain, a bit of puff or, better still, a bit of brown. I knew the familiar trade pattern. So-and-so would have told Jason he could borrow the chairs, meaning they'd be gone as soon as he'd received his fix. Nothing was for keeps, only to secure the next passport to paradise.

Parked sadly in the corner of the room were Jason's few possessions. His CD collection sat in one ragged cardboard box, the flap of one side torn and hanging. A DVD player and various other electrical appliances given for Christmases or birthdays were crammed into two other dishevelled boxes, the leads draping on the carpet like tentacles. Alongside these stood a broken coffee table with a TV perched on top and one of the legs propped up with books and magazines. I noticed the overflowing ashtray balanced alongside and, as I picked it up to empty it, the table wobbled precariously.

A stench of burning food suddenly became overpowering as a plume of smoke was released from the kitchen. Behind the clanging pans, Jason shouted loudly, "I'm cooking breakfast. D'yer want some?"

He was eager to impress me with his culinary skills. Opening the front door to release the smoke, I shouted a loud warning about the fire alarm. Jason jumped to close the oven door he was peering into, sending steam and smoke into his face. I took in the stark image of my bewildered brother standing in the middle of the kitchen, a thick cigar hanging from the side of his mouth. As the smoke dissipated, the cigar resembled a half-cremated sausage, fat oozing from one end and cascading onto his chin and tee-shirt then dripped onto his flapping boot.

I had to smile, noticing the sausage also had two uncooked strips running uniformly down each side making it resemble a stick of rock. If he didn't succeed in incinerating the kitchen, he would most certainly be giving himself a decent bout of e-coli.

Through the haze, his gangly frame took the form of a band conductor poking at his edible orchestra: the exploding sausages, the spitting beans oozing onto the hob, the eggs he stabbed at in the frying pan sending a barrage of oil onto his hand. He released a tirade of expletives at the food he was convinced was conspiring against him. For a crescendo he spun on his heels with a truly impressive act of dexterity, just keeping his balance before rushing towards the grill.

"Shit! The fucking bacon!" Flicking his bedraggled hair from his eyes with a fat splattered finger, he mumbled from the corner of his mouth, "You sure you don't want some?" Staring at the e-coli sausage still miraculously hanging from his mouth, I declined and watched him scoop the various elements onto one gigantic plate of artery-blocking deliciousness. But I laughed under my breath, enjoying his energy.

"It's the anniversary of Diane's death today. A year ago."

Jason sat on the chair opposite me, balancing the food mountain on his spindly knees, looking at me dismally. A typically abrupt transformation, manic to depressed in seconds. As suddenly as he'd reminded me of his dead girlfriend's tragic passing, his elation lay as incinerated as his breakfast.

That's what I'm here for, I reminded myself. Whenever sadness descended on Jason and life conspired against him, I felt it was my duty to try to make him see the point, any point, of helping himself. Eager for him to continue his good work, I reminded him of his aspiration that, once he'd had a few months' rehabilitation, life would take a definitive turn for the better. Could it be possible, I speculated, that he might one day be able to work?

Meanwhile, he shovelled forkfuls of food into his mouth and stared meditatively at his belongings before slinging his empty plate into the sink and lighting another cigarette. His smoke trailed behind him like an ethereal scarf as he pulled the door open and blew it outside, but the place already reeked of fags. With his long coat draped around him, silhouetted in the doorway he resembled a character from a horror movie, gaunt and menacing.

"I hope I get some peace here," he said, looking upstairs.

"Why?" I said. "What are the neighbours like, noisy?"

"It's not the neighbours I'm worried about," Jason said half laughing, half despondent. "I was woken up last night by knocking on my bedroom door."

I glanced towards the kitchen cupboard and thought about his meds, they were supposed to stop these hallucinations.

"You're in a new place, Jason, you don't understand the acoustics yet. Someone knocking next door could easily sound much nearer. They're only thin walls." I tapped one to demonstrate, sounding like a surveyor.

"I'm scared of that bed shaking thing happening again," he admitted fearfully.

Why he had to repeat these stories several times a year was beyond me. I set about the task of throwing his mind a curveball, to steer his thoughts in another direction. I pointed at the TV balancing on the coffee table.

"Maybe we should get this place organised?"

"I'm going to do all that, don't worry." He flicked his cigarette into the ashtray and looked towards the doorway leading to the stairs. "I never want that to happen to again. Frightened the life out of me."

My deflection had failed. He needed to repeat his stories so I didn't forget how his apparitions and hallucinations made him feel, frightened and helpless.

I have a knack of being able to locate my brother, though it's more to do with him being a creature of habit than any sixth sense. The off-licence selling out-of-date cans to struggling alcoholics was only a few hundred yards from the Centre Jason attended – as the nature documentaries Jason watched so keenly always stressed, sharks feed first on easy prey – so it was my first port of call some days later.

Coasting past the shop, I caught site of my brother as an avalanche of rain cascaded against my windscreen. Northerly blasts of deranged wind buffeted the deluge into persistent torrents, and there was my brother walking through it all. The pavement was a series of small lakes and he ploughed through them all oblivious, his open coat flapping, revealing successive layers of wet, unkempt clothing. His partially closed eyes gazed aimlessly. I drove past so I could pull into the side road ahead and pick him up, his inner torment as profoundly tangible as I'd ever seen it.

He'd left a despairing, barely decipherable message on my mobile. The gist was something about another derailed meeting with the psychiatrist accompanied by multiple explanations as to why it had all gone wrong. He sounded afraid that he'd finally cast the death knell on his hopes of ever getting real help in a rehab programme. Despite finally being granted funds to secure his place, the happiness derived from this triumph had been short-lived before his demons came back to torment him with a vengeance.

I parked the car, my heart heavy. Watching my dismantled brother staggering along through the sopping windscreen was like watching a film tragedy you already knew the ending of but you can't turn it off because you're a part of it. And I watched the loony-spotters gawping at him, his presence serving as a shocking reminder of the poor, tortured souls that pass us through life without hope.

Jason stopped dead yards from my car, fumbling frantically in his pockets for his saviour, life's nectar. Pulling out a can, he moved to the dry of the bus shelter on the corner of the side road to enjoy the contents. There, he stared trancelike at the wheels of the passing traffic, listening to the relentless hypnotic swathes of wet ploughing rubber on tarmac. I knew he'd find the sound calming, poetic in its pulse and rhythm. Upending the can he necked the contents, his Adam's Apple bobbing like a yoyo.

I opened the window to get his attention but then changed my mind. Jason was talking convivially to a lone, dark figure he'd seen from the corner of his eye.

"After forty years of having nothing to do with his own son, you'd think he'd at least return my fucking calls." His slurred voice quivered with emotion, a mixture of vehement indignation and hurt he couldn't disguise.

A bus squealed to a halt in front of him, sending a tidal flow of murky water over the curb onto his desecrated leather boots. The pneumatic hiss of the closing door released a passing hoard of strangers, all oblivious to Jason's anguish. He stared at them silently and I felt I could read his mind. 'It's okay for them, they're normal.' Barely glancing at the silent stranger, he continued his monologue.

"I'm past it now anyway. Who wants to know me? I'm a fucking mess. I'm finished. I'm nothing. He should come and see me. He's my Dad." His voice cracked again. I knew he was trying to dissect the previous years, his hopes having been reunited with his father. But their contact had come to a virtual halt. Now he was suffering the pain of rejection all over again.

I knew the way my brother's mind operated, the way his memory could blur from faint recollection to profound and vivid reconstruction. I knew how hard he'd found the initial reunion and how much expectation he'd pinned on it. They'd enjoyed a brief honeymoon during which Jason had withdrawn from heroin and began rejuvenating his life. He'd dared to believe their reunion would cement a lasting relationship, his father would become his saviour and make everything okay.

But the beacon of hope had been extinguished and replaced by further rejection. Now he was having to come to terms with the fact their relationship had come full circle.

What really vexed me was our father's inability to understand

Jason's qualities. Some of my brother's greatest traits were a mirror of Leo's. He was a gifted creative, a talented artist, often disenchanted and always off the wall. The only crucial difference between them was that my brother was overly sensitive and overly generous. Our father never grasped this despite all the months Jason spent in that caravan trying to get to know him.

Now I understood how Jason's love for his father had given him the strength to withdraw from heroin. It was impressive, the unrequited love my brother harboured. Yet despite his efforts to bond and rebuild their relationship, within a few months our father was now keeping him at arm's length.

Perhaps Leo just didn't know what to do with him; it wasn't easy tending to his needs. He'd run out of ideas of how to help his son and I understood that completely. The thing is, though, if you love another person you just keep on trying regardless. That was something more than he could muster. Jason took this second rejection badly.

I continued watching him sitting on the corner seat at the bus stop, shaking his head and considering himself as a nothing.

"Sorry mate," he continued. "I'm going on. I'm just lonely at the moment. Not mad. Maybe just a bit crazy, but definitely not mad. There's nothing wrong with wanting to have someone is there? If not my Dad, then a good woman would be nice." He smiled, no doubt remembering Diane.

I observed him glancing at the silent figure beside him indignantly, hoping for some sign of kinship or friendliness, then there was an uncomfortable silence as my brother's eyes confirmed what I could already see for myself. An overwhelming look of consternation returned to Jason as he looked again at the dark, silent stranger. It was, in fact, a discarded and dishevelled umbrella.

I called out to him and he climbed into my car, looking wounded by his display of absurdity, then proceeded to explain how the morning had been a complete disaster.

When he'd finally turned up to his appointment with the psychiatrist, he was forty minutes late. Jason knew the meeting was important and could decide his fate with the rehabilitation centre, the focus of his future hopes. He had to attend this meeting on his own and I'd given him a rousing talking-to in preparation. Although I only had Jason's best intentions at heart, it later worried me that perhaps I'd left his mind in a chaotic spiral of hopeful possibilities.

"This is the big one. You've got to give it a go. Last chance. It's worth a try. You might make some friends, even a girlfriend."

Unfortunately, he hadn't been able to repress the demon taunting his mind that morning when he awoke. He was possessed with a burning desire for one last indulgence before he was committed, a last descent into drug-induced comfort and obliteration before he finally faced reality.

He'd rationalised that he had plenty of time before the meeting so had walked a mile to an estate he knew well; it was his most successful haunt whenever he needed Class A. Standing in the urine-drenched basement of a dirty, partly burnt-out tower block, he'd waited anxiously, fidgeting with the solitary note in his pocket, his last tenner. He waited and watched for someone he recognised who could provide for his insatiable need. In the partial darkness, a figure entered through the partly boarded and graffitied entrance.

The embittered character immediately noticed Jason and there was a brief exchange of eye contact. Silence. The body language was uncertain between them, but each understood their separate agendas. After the deal was done, suddenly and without a word, the tall, dark and unkempt stranger – partially supported by an NHS crutch and wielding a walking stick – attacked the druggie standing in front of him in the urine-stained concrete basement.

"Jason, are you honestly trying to tell me that you're late for our meeting because you were mugged by a disabled man?"

The psychiatrist was understandably angry and frustrated. He'd heard the impossible stories and excuses for lateness and absence many times from too many hapless patients. Despite Jason's welling tears and protestations of truth, the man was having none of it. Jason's chances of free rehab to change the direction of his life were dissolving rapidly. He also understood that he was ultimately responsible for this disaster, the innocent victim of what he needed rescuing from.

He'd looked at the psychiatrist with dislike. He hated most of these young medical professionals with a passion anyway. To them, he was a laboratory gerbil, an experiment in progress. How could they know about his real life at all? They were all manufactured in a university without any comprehension of how life really was for someone like him. The man didn't know anything about his suffering and his struggles with addiction.

Frustratingly for Jason, there was another conundrum. How could he begin to tell this uncaring shrink that he believed his deceased girlfriend Diane was trying to communicate with him from beyond the grave? Would he believe or even accept that he'd started hearing other things around the house? He was just a pen pusher, he couldn't understand that world.

"Look, I've got no money. No drugs."

Jason stood and turned his pockets out, desperate, his hands upturned. As if my brother's pleading innocence and empty pockets were ever going to cut the mustard. The psychiatrist had watched my brother disbelievingly. Shaking his head, he gave an infuriating and ill-concealed tut of contempt as he returned to his clipboard, scribbling his notes on the desk with conviction.

Jason felt he'd been judged, tried and sentenced. But most of all, he felt dislike emanating from this man, and it made him feel angry. In my car, he scrunched his fist into a bony ball, as uncharacteristic fantasies of aggression flicked though his mind.

"I've got principles," he insisted. "I'm not violent, Marc, you know that."

Still, he well knew that he couldn't display anger to a psychiatrist, any outburst would resign him to the druggie dustbin for eternity. He'd watched the man bitterly, wondering how much more arrogant intolerance and rejection he could actually endure. 'Fucking robot,' he thought, but managed to maintain his composure despite the frustration and anger eating away at him.

Shaking his head slowly, the psychiatrist had let out a protracted sigh.

"I'm struggling to know what to do with you, Jason. You're too irritable to talk to today."

Feeling a shot of indignation pass through him, Jason said nothing. He contemplated leaving the Centre and just going home so he could obliterate the pain and humiliation with a wrap of tranquility that would transport him to that magical quiet place he knew so well. He had started to trust and confide in his Care Worker, Trish, before she'd left the Centre, but now he'd been left this unfeeling moron.

"We have concluded you're not schizophrenic, Jason," the psychiatrist pronounced without looking up, tapping the notes with his pen.

"I know I'm not fucking mad. I've told you that." Jason felt a warming defiance, wondering who the 'we' really were and whether what they thought really mattered at all.

"I'll put in a recommendation with the Rehabilitation Centre and we'll see what they say. It's not easy to get fully sponsored places, you know the costs are considerable." He was more than a little patronising as he looked at my brother.

Jason had simply nodded, wishing he could talk to someone else about his troubles. He detested anyone he perceived as looking down on him. Feeling unfulfilled after enduring this further bout of probing and form-filling, without getting a chance to tell his side of the story, he was in despair. The empty pointlessness of such sessions resounded in his mind. Surely there must be someone else who will listen like Trish did.

Feeling like he wanted to either cry or maybe even die, but unsure which option would be best, he'd thought about just leaving the interview. He'd thought about going home and what he would do once he got there. But then, he was also acutely aware that, every time he escaped the world, coming back again was so much harder.

I parked the car outside his place and tried to pacify his obvious irritation about the meeting, his life trajectory and his hatred of the world in general.

"It's just been a bad day, Jason. You must keep going so you can get into rehab. You've been doing well."

"I know I've got to try but they just don't want to help me. They think I'm a piece of shit." Jason began crying, his eyes red and as raw as his emotions. He hated being considered a parasite. "They don't believe anything I tell them." He produced a clod of damp tissues and blew his nose hard, trying to stem his sobs.

"You can talk to me, Jason. You know I always listen. Even if I don't want to." I smiled and gave him a friendly shove. He tried to see the funny side and then his tears stopped and he began to explain what was on his mind as we walked across the road and he opened his front door.

Diane had been knocking on his door at night. Her soft, deliberate knock: two knocks in close succession followed by a pause and then another knock, the knock she'd always used before entering the flat they'd shared. It was unmistakably Diane.

The trouble was, Jason was the boy who cried wolf. He'd fucked things up so much in the past with these so-called professionals, with his claims of ludicrous happenings and the strange things he believed he saw. Now he felt these cold, clinical experts perceived him as a joke and a hopeless crank, balancing precariously between sanity and lunacy.

So why bother anymore? They didn't believe anything he said. He had given up trying. It was better to escape for a few hours or maybe a day, to meander among his mountain of prescription drugs, a chase of heroin or even a dozen strong ciders. Anything was better than looking into the faces of people who think you're a nothing, just something to be pitied rather than understood.

His mind was switching between his hope for a free chance at rehab and the knowledge that he was going to blast his senses again. For a while he wouldn't feel anything, he would be neither happy nor sad. Numb was the best feeling.

"She always comes when I'm at my saddest," Jason explained,

When the door to his home swung open with a reluctant squeal, we surveyed the carnage from earlier: the cans on the carpet, the ashtray balancing on the speaker which lay face down on the floor, ash festooning the carpet and sheets of newspaper leading to the foot of the stairs. This was normal order for him. He immediately began picking up the debris, tidying the newspapers away before taking the ashtray to the overflowing bin in the kitchen.

In his own individual way, Jason was quite organised. If he'd walked through the front door into the tiny living room and the stained two-seater sofa was on the other side of the room, he'd assume he must have moved it himself. If the television was left on, he knew he would have simply forgotten to turn it off before leaving. This was normal organic chaos for him. The constant apparent disorder reflected his emotional wellbeing.

What overwhelmed Jason in the house were the small things, the details only he knew about, and of course Diane. He had his quirks, his obsessive-compulsive tendencies, but no-one knew about them except her.

Now, inside the kitchen, Jason had stopped abruptly. He analysed the unfamiliar arrangement on the sink. Two teaspoons were sitting on the drainer, the cups of the spoons pointing upwards, the spoons in the shape of a cross. His mind abruptly stopped cartwheeling. He always placed the spoons cup down and horizontal. It was a kind of religious act, a ceremony and a code of practice he never deviated from.

No, this was a communication as definite as a visual apparition itself. Through all the mess, carnage and toil of his mind, it presented itself perfectly as undeniable proof.

Diane sends her love.

16

REHAB

The traffic whooshed along the one-way system as I cupped my ear to the Reception speaker and pressed the buzzer to the Rehabilitation Centre. A distinct rumble warned of another impending summer shower. But despite the melancholy skies, I felt full of optimism.

Jason had finally begun his first days of rehab. Years of petitioning had been rewarded and now, after five days inside the walls, I was going to see him beginning his second shot at life. What wasn't certain was what long-term plan and itinerary the wellbeing team had in mind for Jason; he'd understood this was an initial trial to see how well he handled being institutionalised. It was a prelude to, potentially, a full-term rehabilitation place of three or possibly six months and a greater chance of correcting the habits of more than three decades of self-abuse.

This was a new day in the same town for my brother, but a day I hoped to look back on in the future with the luxury of nostalgia.

Looking above the gate at the white, sterile building, dancing clouds floated across the large mirrored windows facing the town centre. Inside I was bubbling with excitement and curiosity. I'd never been inside the place before, or any other similar kind of institution. This was a first for both of us.

It was over five days since I'd seen Jason. He was now halfway through his initial stint, adding to my apprehension about how I'd find him on the other side of the walls. It may not seem like something to celebrate, but this was the longest period in decades that he'd been off everything. Mindful of this, I figured there was a fair chance I'd be able to gauge the outcome of any longer-term treatment, should it be offered. I narrowed my brother's current state of mind to two likely options: stir crazy or straighter than he'd been in decades and practically a stranger.

Finally, a puritanical voice answered the entrance buzzer. I told the robot my name and who I was visiting and was answered by the lock opening to the inadequate-looking gate.

There were many rumours circulating about the Centre's efficiency, or lack of it. Below the small residential facility was a Day Centre with a café, a well-known meeting place for people who were simply playing and abusing the system. These rumours fuelled Jason's initial scepticism about taking up the offer of a residency there. He referred to the place as The Slippery, as in the slippery slope. But he'd been reassured that it was better than many facilities and he'd not be sharing his time with sentenced criminals just looking for chances to skip a prison sentence. That was one of his major concerns.

It was well known that many troubled souls attending the Day Centre collected free syringes or Methadone prescriptions before migrating to the surrounding parks to score a real hit, trading their medications and supplies for cash. A narcotic supplies swap shop. As this was regarded as a good place for free handouts, dealers and users alike travelled for miles to take advantage of this easy symbiosis. Dealers preyed on users, hanging around the building and surrounding green spaces. Users found the temptation to score irresistible with such a plentiful supply of tradable paraphernalia available. It wasn't hard to secure Nirvana if you knew where to go. And naturally, the local schools weren't happy about the close proximity of the Centre.

I entered, battling many preconceptions. Reaching the corner of the second flight of steps, a plume of cigarette smoke greeted me. Above, the bonhomie sounds of laughter and friendly conversation accompanied the sweet smell of Golden Virginia. The unmistakable odour was accompanied by the unmistakable voice of my brother.

I stood and listened, trying to determine how many others were with him, perhaps three female voices along with two men. A ripple of laughter spread among them. Hesitantly, I climbed another step like some sleuth detective and heard Jason start one of his favourite parables.

"Of course, they didn't really land on the moon. That's just what they want us to believe." Quintessentially my brother.

By the lull in the laughter and conversation it was evident the crew he was hanging with were intrigued by what this enigmatic character had to say. Jason had returned to his affable, quizzical self again. A fresh rush of optimism swept over me.

At the top of the stairs I stood at a distance from the group, surreptitiously watching them from the stairwell. They sat in the corner opposite the entrance to the Centre on a small patio. I stood unobserved, like a ghost, smiling to myself. Jason sat fervently inhaling a cigarette, smiling profusely at two attractive young women sitting next to him. Things were definitely looking up.

Another woman with her back to me contemplated her steely blue cigarette smoke drifting out towards the river, making occasional comments over her shoulder. Two men talking just inside the doorway flicked cigarette ash into a tray attached to the wall, and one of them tapped my brother on the shoulder to offer him some cigarette papers. There was a tangible camaraderie. They remained oblivious as I stood observing them like an explorer might a lost tribe, wondering what ritual they'd perform next.

One of the girls was a mischievous-looking blonde wearing a white puffer jacket. She gazed dizzily at Jason, smiling and clearly enthralled by everything he had to say on all matters conspiracy theory. During moments of stillness, she inhaled hard on her cigarette like it was the only thing she'd ever wanted. My brother's stories were followed by hilarity and the pattern repeated. I watched the motley crew's laughter ripple around them.

Jason had an audience and for once it wasn't a crowd of faceless onlookers staring at a freak show. I'd never seen him like this before. This disjointed clan were like-minded souls emerging from various stages of dependency, sharing a brief interlude from their troubles. Intermittently their smiles slid, the only clue to their inner turmoil. It was warming to see the troubled souls revelling in each other's company, united by their quest for sobriety, life's tortures briefly forgotten.

I walked towards them wondering how I'd be greeted, an intruding outsider after all. As Jason began another story, the two girls stopped laughing and glanced up at me. They viewed me with suspicion and timid curiosity. Then Jason turned, his eyes proclaiming surprise and pleasure simultaneously.

"Blimey. You made me jump." He patted his heart then winked and smiled at the girls again. He'd become quite the entertainer. "This is my brother, Marc," he declared with the utmost satisfaction. The two men just inside the doorway peered out from the darkness like tortoises and waved hello before disappearing back inside. "Thanks for coming to see me, Marc," Jason beamed.

It was like entering the realms of some surreal dream, seeing him so affable and entirely together. I smiled at the group. Grinning happily, the corners of his eyes crinkled like eagle's claws. He stood slowly and combed his hair through with his hands, the dark nicotine stains on his smoking fingers contrasting with his freshly shaven complexion.

"This is Georgia, and that's Alison," he said.

I put my hand out to the two girls, shaking Georgia's limp fingers with an immediate rush of empathy. Alison awkwardly put her hand up to greet mine with similar fragility, coupled with misplaced suspicion.

"We've been hearing all about you," Georgia said, smiling.

I speculated what intimacies my brother could have shared

with his chums and if any of them could be incriminating. As I nodded meekly at Georgia and Alison, to my further discomfort they burst into another fit of unexplained laughter. I felt awkward, remembering the old pictures of me at our mother's house, such as the one of me watering the garden wearing nothing but a pair of wellies when I was three.

It occurred to me that their hilarity probably had nothing to do with me, but the concoctions of happy pills prescribed by the institution to placate inmates. Whatever they prescribed appeared to be working. I wondered how much of their carefree happiness could be attributed, though, to them experiencing sobriety and camaraderie for the first time.

Jason stopped laughing and pointed towards the smoking girl in the corner.

"That's Sue," he said.

The girl nodded, scanning me cynically. She walked past the other girls without eye contact and made her way into the Centre. Alison huddled on her chair pulling up the lapels on her jacket to shield her from the strengthening wind. Then without warning the clouds emptied shards of rain, splattering the communal smoking area and sending the girls screeching like seagulls into the sanctuary of the open doorway.

"Come in, I'll show you around, Marc." Jason spoke with a hint of pride. "I'll introduce you to the others." He walked confidently through the door as behind me another ominous rumble of thunder growled in the distance.

"Do I need to sign in?" I asked, surprised it was all so casual. I hadn't phoned to say I was coming although Jason's key worker had told him that family could visit after he'd settled in.

"No, it's cool, Marc. You're my brother."

Jason strolled inside confidently. I felt suspicious of his liberal approach to the security and made my way towards the entrance expecting an inquisition. Inside, I was surprised to find clean, freshly painted high walls, broken by expansive skylights above. The perfume of home-cooked food permeated. Jason guided me down a corridor punctuated by open doors, each one illuminating the hallway with daylight. The weird mix of homeliness and institutional efficiency wasn't entirely unpleasant.

"They like us to keep our room doors open during the day," Jason informed me over his shoulder, pointing to a doorway ahead. "That's my room at the end on the right. I've got my own TV and everything." He spoke with contented enthusiasm.

I peeked inside and found it pristine and ordered, his khaki jacket draped over a chair, his few belongings on a small table. The perfectly made single bed completing the room's fresh and cleanliness. Jason turned and walked towards an even brighter burst of light entering the corridor.

The communal sitting room contained soft furniture, settees, armchairs and scatter cushions with a bookshelf at the far end. Inside were several more unfamiliar faces, some of whom looked notably bemused by their new sobriety like children making fresh discoveries. Jason stood in the centre of the room and began making introductions.

"This is David."

He gestured towards a man in his mid-thirties, perched on the plush brown leather sofa dividing the room. He glanced up and said hello then continued preparing his next roll-up. Wearing a grey polo-neck jumper, brown cords and dark-brown loafers, David looked smart and together like a teacher. I felt unsure where he fitted into the group. He finished rolling his cigarette and walked towards me with the brisk efficiency of a soldier, putting his hand out.

"Hello, Marc. I'm Dave, resident psychiatrist here at the Centre." He cast his hand about him as if spreading a spell across the other inmates. I shook his hand politely. Then without warning, he began hacking a syrupy smoker's laugh, unnerving me with its spontaneity. Jason placed a hand on his shoulder with surprising familiarity and giggled.

"He's one of us, Marc. He's just having a laugh, aren't you, Dave?"

"You gave me away, you bugger." Dave shook his head, still battling his syrupy hack. "I had you going there, didn't I, Marc?"

"You did indeed, Dave. If that's your real name." I put my hands up surrendering with a friendly nod.

From a small room adjoined to the communal lounge, I noticed a dark-haired woman sitting in a leather swivel chair and smiling. She made her way over. Mid- to late-thirties, I estimated, motherly and likeable.

"Very nice to meet you. I'm Sandra," she said softly. "Feel free to use the dining room if you want some privacy. Dinner isn't for an hour or so." Sandra motioned towards another room with sliding French doors.

"Thanks Sandra, you're a diamond!" Jason smirked. Again it struck me as my brother spoke how at home and confident he already was in his new environment. His familiarity with the other inmates and staff alike was a strict contrast to his previous incarnation less than a week ago. When he'd agreed to his admittance, tearful and full of trepidation, he'd issued me a clear warning.

"I'll give it a go, Marc. But I'm telling you, if I don't like it I'm leaving after a day. I don't want to be around a load of fucking smack and pissheads."

"You've spent your whole life doing that, Jace," was my obvious retort. "At least this lot are trying to get clean."

His hands were shaking as he tried lighting his cigarette that day, mostly through fear. But now it was as if he'd been there for months, not days. I was experiencing a juxtaposition – now I was the stranger feeling awkward and out of place.

He led me through the open-plan kitchen where a couple were preparing ingredients on an ample worktop. I marvelled at the lack of disorder or chaos; it just wasn't what I'd been expecting. We walked through the glass doors into the bright airy dining room, stopping to take in the view through the wall of windows. The sky was split between grey storm clouds and promising streaks of blue. The window provided a view of the town, where busy shoppers and bustling traffic continued obliviously.

Jason sat across from me at the communal dining table facing the window, the filtering light against the clinical white walls casting a celestial glow behind him. The room was quiet, only convivial sounds from the kitchen audible.

"How have you been then, mate?" I looked into his eyes, trying to interpret his thoughtful expression.

"Yeah… it's been good. Really nice group I'm with."

His voice started to crack slightly with the emotion of his experience. For the first time since we were children, here was my brother in his most uncontaminated state. The boy I'd gradually lost sight of during childhood was now a slightly puzzled man. Holding my gaze, Jason's piercing blue eyes illuminated his bewilderment at life's sadness, the reflection of the cityscape and changing clouds animated within them. He didn't need to explain his feelings, I read them with clarity.

"So you're happy to finally be on the wagon, then?" I asked.

His eyes welled as a cascade of tears splashed onto the table. His gaze was fixed on the world behind, the perilous world of reality. When he was like this it was easy to imagine him standing in the garden in Sussex, hiding and making camps within the labyrinths of vegetation. The hope I'd held for decades was becoming real. Finally, Jason would be healed. I allowed myself to believe this, cautiously remembering it was still early days.

Had these first few days of lucidity given him a fresh perspective on living a different life? He'd confronted his fears and already spent time in contemplation. Maybe he was now pondering how he'd redeem the remainder of his life. That would bewilder anyone. Jason had already learned something important, that people liked him and enjoyed his company. To his amazement he could converse with others without being under the influence.

"Maybe I'm not that weird and fucked up after all?" he said, wiping away the small puddle with his sleeve.

"This could be the making of you, Jace. You could be clean. You might even find a girlfriend!" I concentrated on the perks of rehab with another cheeky smile. "Your two friends are nice."

My brother grinned, the tobacco stains on his teeth a reminder of his journey, his hidden turmoil still festering behind the emotion in his eyes. He shook his head.

"I want to be normal. I've been so fucking lonely. I've actually enjoyed being here with other people. I didn't think that would happen."

"That's great. You're already looking a lot healthier."

Jason's eyes dried and his face became less pensive as his melancholy released.

"It's great not being alone at night. Talking to someone until I'm tired enough to sleep. I've been sleeping like a baby in here." Whatever it was that was still bugging him behind the surface lifted and I began to feel upbeat again.

"So what normally happens during the course of a day? Do you have group sessions and share life stories?" I felt anxious for him, that once he had a willing audience what stories he'd tell and how they'd be perceived. It was a familiar dread I'd grown used to when he spoke to care workers and psychiatrists and spontaneously blurt out outrageous statements without warning.

"Yeah. We spend hours doing group talks and discussion." Jason frowned wearily. "They've let me keep my prescription drugs, my Haloperidol." He pulled out a pouch of tobacco and some papers and, with every ounce of concentration, began creating what he clearly hoped would be his most perfectly created roll-up to date.

"What's that got to do with your group sessions?" I asked.

Jason finished making his cigarette and admired it between his nicotine-stained fingers.

"The other night, the support worker saw my legs jumping when we were in a group meeting. He pulled me out of my group to give me a drugs test. Wanker!"

"Surely they must know about your meds?" I asked, shocked that this could be overlooked.

"They had a list of my meds but this guy didn't know about

them. I had to tell him what I was taking and what effect it had before he'd let me back in. He was well out of order."

It was disheartening to see Jason's outrage at being made to feel like a freak in front of others. I felt a need to defuse things.

"Well, if he didn't know about it, it's a bit disappointing but forgivable, yeah?" Still smarting, Jason didn't register my logic. "Anyway, have you had any further conversations with lovely psychiatrists?" I continued, trying to add a bit of humour. Jason just eyed me suspiciously.

"Yeah. Just before they let me come here. I saw the one from the Centre again. I can't pronounce his name. He asked me about the voices I hear and the things that I see. He was a total wanker as usual."

As Jason told me this, apprehension threw its coils around me like a python.

"I also told him the other psychiatrist had already said I wasn't schizophrenic. They did all these assessments. Remember me telling you?" I nodded and Jason shrugged. "Mind you, the shrink did also say he thought I was fucking mad." Jason laughed self-deprecatingly. I tried to work out the logic of this, watching his anger turn to laughter so seamlessly.

"What did you tell them about the voices?"

Prior to entering rehab he'd been in no fit state to discuss the full extent of his manifestations. Paranoia gripped me further. Maybe the system was just getting him clean enough to turn on him, thinking he was another mass murderer in the making.

"I told them that sometimes the voices tell me to kill. But I always ignore them. I told them I've been followed by something all my life."

"Shit!"

I looked around the room with fresh dismay. Jason's honesty was often his worst enemy, and my naïve hope that rehabilitation would quickly ease his visions and psychosis was unravelling. I recalled my past mindset when I'd given serious thought to having him sectioned. Considering these latest facts it seemed probable the mental health team were already ahead of me.

"Sorry, but it's true." Jason read my exasperation. "I do sometimes hear that, but I'd never do anything. I just block it out. You know I'm not violent. I've never been violent."

Thankfully, this was an undeniable truth otherwise I'm sure we'd have been contemplating a lengthy spell in some dank, depressing mental institution. Logic decreed he wouldn't have been allowed into this place if he'd been perceived as a danger to others. But I felt the direction of Jason's future care was still balanced precariously.

"What did they say when you told them that?"

"They said that when I get out of here, the police might come and talk to me about it. They just kept asking me about it over and over again. It really pissed me off."

I gathered my thoughts. I'd been premature in hoping for too much too soon. Jason's deep belief that some entity follows him everywhere wasn't going to cease overnight. Yet I had to believe it would eventually.

"So how was it left, Jason? They let you come in here, didn't they? That's a good sign."

"There was another psychiatrist who came in and talked with me. He said that my head might clear after a few weeks in rehab." This may all be a test, I rationalised, yet there was evidence the mental health team held hope his psychosis would clear. It's an unavoidable fact that the process of rehabilitation is slow and precarious and sometimes appears like an impossible dream.

"I don't really understand. You look well. You've not had any drink or drugs. You're lucid. Are you still trying to tell me you're tormented by spirits?" I looked at him apologetically. I'd said what I was thinking out loud and now he looked at me with despair. He could see that he'd let me down.

"I know it's hard to understand," he appealed. "You think I've just ruined my life with drugs and drink but I know what really happens." Occasionally, whenever Jason shared his madness, I had entertained the ludicrous: could something unfathomable really have followed and tormented him since childhood? I felt the possibility of maintaining rational conversation dissolve, my earlier optimism blighted.

"So when do you get out?"

"They said I can go at the end of the week. I'm going to a few meetings with Steve, the guy that did a talk here yesterday evening. He's a good guy, Steve. He's been there and now he's recovered."

I had to wonder where Steve had actually been and if it was anywhere as dark as my brother's experiences.

"Steve sounds good," I said, trying to sound chipper. Then a ridiculous thought entered my head like lightning: did Steve even exist?

Jason left rehab after ten days and received only two follow-up meetings before his care worker told him she didn't need to see him anymore. Did they think he was cured? He didn't get an answer. Jason was as dumbfounded and disenchanted as I was with the mental health system. He'd weaned himself off heroin without professional help, so he believed he could manage without further rehabilitation as long as he had his meds.

The downward spiral began afresh.

It was a late morning in September when I entered Jason's one-bedroom home. I'd not heard from him for many days and was concerned. I'd deliberated hard about entering with the spare key, feeling uncertain of what I'd find – perhaps a clue to my brother's whereabouts, if not he himself in some intoxicated and vulnerable state.

Pushing open the front door, I stood in the small lounge full of uneasiness I couldn't contain. I felt nauseous, and not just because of the putrid smell emanating from the kitchen bin. Where was he? The television was on but there was no sound. The BBC newsflash across the bottom of the screen told of a murder nearby. The floor and bay window ledge were littered with empty cans and bottles. It hadn't taken long for my brother to fall back into bad habits.

The ashtray on top of the TV was overflowing. The butts were cold, no smoke, no life. On the floor, an open newspaper had been repeatedly written on with exaggerated handwriting in my brother's hand, emboldening the scrawl so it was thick and menacing, almost loud. The words 'Fuck Me' covered most of the pages. Underneath was a small annotation, a figure that looked vaguely female. I found it confusing.

"Jason. Are you here, Jace?"

Walking into the kitchen, I opened the fridge. The milk was out of date. A half-open packet of bacon and a single egg box were the only other contents. I ran through the evidence in the house again like a forensic detective.

"Jason. Jason, are you about?" My voice reverberated with a dull, empty echo. Silence was the only reply.

In the sink was a single plate and several items of cutlery, unwashed. Empty frozen food boxes, microwavable delicacies labelled Meal for One were scattered randomly along the tiny worktop. It made me feel dejected and tearful.

"Jason. Are you there?"

Looking around the downstairs living room for further clues, I hoped desperately Jason would just walk through the door or come down the stairs. Outside, rushing traffic proclaimed the indifference of daily life. Two women were talking outside accompanied by the rumble of pushchair wheels fading into the distance. Bus brakes squealed and the heavy hydraulic doors hissed open, reminding me how easily others' lives continues regardless of yours and of those you love.

The silence inside forced me to venture upstairs. At the foot, I detected a small scrap of lined paper on the floor near the first step, a note that simply said 'Diane' on the top. The other words were faded and indecipherable.

As I climbed, the noxious smell from the bin hanging in

the air, I looked back at the degradation and tried reminding myself of happier times. I spotted the picture on the wall that I'd taken of my brother on the fire escape outside my office, his face bathed in golden sunshine. He was sober and almost happy that day, I remembered, his blue eyes reflecting the day's brightness. Then I laughed out loud as I remembered finding him in a complete state of dilapidation once, trying to hoover my office one morning… without a hoover. What else was I to do? It was horribly humorous, seeing the looks on the faces of my speechless staff.

On the upstairs landing the carpet was worn and dirty. I remembered my fearful brother telling me he heard scratching and noises that disturbed him at night from the outside wall, that something was trying to get at him. I wondered what it all meant to him, the things he swore that moved in his bedroom, the orbs, the voices and other manifestations.

The door to the bathroom was open, displaying the lurid pink suite, Jason's discarded army greens hanging over the basin. Below, a worn brown leather boot, sole unhinged, and two socks discarded erratically, one draping over the open toilet bowl, the other in the middle of the floor.

"Jason. Are you here?" Silence.

Inside the bathroom I noticed a tin of shaving foam in the bathtub. On the cabinet mirror was the residue of a finger drawing, an image inscribed at some point when the steam from the sink had risen. The image looked like a face, faintly female but unrecognisable. Disturbing. I could almost replay Jason staring into the mirror, his finger carving the steam, his red eyes lucid in the clear marks as torment stared back at him.

The last place to look was the place I least wanted to go. It was the last place he could be, if he was here at all. I knew my brother's bedroom would protest his tragedy, his inability to function, the grime and random carelessness of everything around him.

The bedroom door was partially closed, held ajar by two empty CD cases open on the turquoise-carpeted floor. *Voodoo Child* and

Harvest. I smiled as I remembered listening to *Heart of Gold* by Neil Young with my brother in a happier interlude. The door creaked open. The curtain was partly drawn and a dusty shaft of muted light illuminated the bed. The blankets were crumpled at one end.

Jason was lying face up on the blue sheet, without movement, without consciousness. Headphones hung from his ears but the iPod was silent.

"Jason!" I shouted as I pushed his shoulder.

He didn't stir. That's it, I thought to myself, he's finally managed it. I stared at his lifelessness shape before shaking him with both hands.

Then, as despair surged through me, I noticed movement, a faint flicker of his eyelids. Jason attempted to lift his head with a few short bursts of movement before relaxing into his pillow and eventually opening his eyes to take in his surroundings. He blinked at me fearfully before rolling over with a muffled groan. Turning back to face me sharply there was a look of disorientation and terror on his face.

In his hand, a blade flashed in the filtered window light. My brother thrust the knife blindly in my direction. A discarded pillow on the floor provided a suitable shield and I smothered the blade. On his second attempt to lunge, I seized his arm, twisted it hard and making the weapon drop to the floor with a hollow thud.

"What the fuck are you doing?" I shouted.

I pinned Jason's arms hard against his chest, holding him still until he looked up at me with recognition and with terror, utterly mortified at his terrible mistake.

17

WHO CARES?

After his short stay in rehab, Jason's old habits returned as steadily as the shifting tides of the sea. Crack and coke were the main culprits. Believing there was no hope anymore, he progressively lost belief that he could ever be anything, let alone straight. Five years of struggle transpired. Five years of encouraging him not to give up. During these years, Jason petitioned the Centre for help.

Now he was facing another new challenge. Employment.

It always made me nervous on the day of his appointments to find him manic and irascible. On this particular occasion I found him busy on his doorstep telling the pigeons on his roof to fuck off. The evidence was as clear as the sky above that Jason's meeting with the employment people was going to be a disaster. Even on a good day these things were precarious. I sensed I'd soon be burying my head in my hands, despairing and muttering under my breath, "For fuck's sake, Jason."

He shook his fist at the birds parading on the edge of the guttering, as though they alone were responsible for his woes and heartaches. I admired their indifference to this adversity; if only my brother had the same fortitude.

The notion of phoning to cancel his appointment occurred to me, but then what would I offer as an excuse? He's got pigeon problems? It was going to be a disaster I couldn't avoid, was my dismal conclusion. I was committed, and what else would Jason occupy the morning with? The meeting would be the lesser of two unproductive evils.

I had some small reason for optimism, however. He smelled as though he'd had a bath, a promising sign. The scent of Tesco's Value Soap and that weird cologne my aunt from Norfolk had bought him for Christmas radiated powerfully.

He had also put on his favourite floral collarless shirt, a Christmas present I'd given him several years ago, which was clean and still in relatively good shape. For added formality, he'd taken time to button up both the cuffs and top button, so the shirt looked like it was strangling the blood supply to his skinny neck. His attempt at neatness was stifling him, fuelling my concern about the volatility of his mood. But for the moment I parked my anxiety about the possible long-term side effects of inhaling the chemical grade aftershave.

Standing in the doorway, he admired the shirt and his own uncharacteristic neatness. Arms angled rigidly at his sides, he looked ready for take-off. I studied him in the way I'd done most of my life, acknowledging that, in his own unstable way, Jason was actually dressed for business.

"Do I look smart, Marc? People say I look like John Lennon when I wear this shirt."

"Perhaps, Jason, if I *imagine* hard enough," I answered, trying to visualise him with round tinted glasses. He had the good grace to laugh self-deprecatingly.

"Yeah. Good one. In your dreams, you mean. With your eyes tight shut, eh?"

He padded back into the room to collect his keys and, undoubtedly, to neck the remnants of the cider tin perched on top of the TV. Even in my dreams Jason couldn't look like John Lennon, but I understood that he needed an ego boost that morning more than he needed another tin of cider. He was nervous, his mind twitchy and desperate to lose itself in minor distractions. I had to produce a compliment. It didn't matter if it was small, but it had to be something to communicate with his inner fragility and heal his lack of confidence. A simple compliment was often the magic catalyst to stabilise his mood.

"Well done for making the effort, Jace." I gave his shirt collar a tug and praised him for being clean and tidy. "You look really smart." I stored the facetious joke I had bubbling on the tip of my tongue about needing to phone the water board to explain the sudden increase in his water usage. No, it wasn't actually much of a joke.

Travelling across London by public transport wasn't easy and was expensive and I feared him attempting to cycle down the main roads, so I drove him to appointments. Sod the parking charges, at least he'd get to his appointments safely, albeit not always soundly. If Jason didn't keep his appointments he'd ultimately receive even less support.

And that support was becoming ever more sparse with all the spending cuts to social care. Many health and support services had already been dropped or withdrawn and the tide was well and truly conspiring against the infirm and the fragile. People like Jason. More than at any other time, it was becoming clear that if you didn't, or couldn't, help yourself, there was no help at all.

Like panning for gold, I clung to the small glimmer of hope being offered by this latest group of support workers. Once again I believed that if we kept on panning we'd hit the jackpot and see a better future for Jason.

Over the previous months he'd fretfully considered the remainder of his working years and what he could do to redeem them. His recognition of his squandered time couldn't have been easy to contemplate, looking at the craggy, middle-aged face staring back at him in the mirror. At some point during these reflections, Jason formed an aspiration, something he'd not done since his late teens during his Fine Art Foundation Course. He'd formed a goal but was anxious about trying to make it a reality in case he suffered another debilitating knockback. Jason processed failure as personal rejection. His real fear was that, if he failed, he'd be back to where he started, which was nowhere at all and then he might not bother trying to pick himself up again.

Jason wanted to become a drugs counsellor. He believed, looking at his reflection, that he would be a fine candidate to warn others of where drug and alcohol abuse could lead.

I understood his doubts about attempting this. He doubted he was worthy to become anything in the first place and needed constant inspiration. My well-meaning encouragement was one thing he could count on; what he needed more was encouragement from the social workers and counsellors, those who could pave the way. So far, though, on his search for purpose, he'd met only apathy. Social workers didn't have time for his pipe dreams, they were too under-resourced.

Watching the cogs of his mind turn over his aspiration was like watching an inventor having an eureka moment. Deciding he could do something worthwhile by exposing his own mistakes was a huge realisation. For the first time in decades, I felt a surge of pride in my brother. By becoming a drugs counsellor he could do something selflessly to benefit others and was excited by the prospect. Behind the sometimes nihilist hell-bent on self-destruction lurked a kind-hearted, considerate human being.

"It's hard confronting reality, Marc." Articulating this was slow and ponderous for him, but I pushed him to try. "Everything's an impossible maze after spending thirty-odd years existing in a blur," he explained. Facing the world afresh, he was like a child needing everything explained and the idea of work was a daunting but earnest prospect. "Sometimes I just want to go back to my drug haze on the other side of reality. I know that world better."

I understood how he was caught in the middle of no-man's land. For some, religion bridges the gap; for those without faith, the drive of purpose becomes life's cushion. My feeling of pride in Jason was blighted by the knowledge his new-found purpose would mean parading himself as a living example of what not to do with your life.

The Trust we were going to was an international charity with over two hundred locations. It had primarily been set up to help disadvantaged and disabled people struggling to get back to work. It also claimed it could help people like Jason, who sat on the periphery of that demographic, those wanting to work who were debilitated mentally.

On appointment days my task was to keep Jason positive and his anxiety at bay, which would otherwise make him skittish and unable to present himself clearly to his interviewer. His awkwardness was simply the chaotic way he coped with stressful situations, but an interviewer could easily consider him uncooperative or, worse still, unemployable.

Increasingly, Jason was facing the discomfort of these face-to-face meetings with the rawness of sobriety. He dreaded the notion of being judged and graded as a person. His lack of confidence of ever being able to cut the mustard among the working nation was a contributory factor to his suffocating hopelessness. Paranoia goaded him, making him succumb to the fear that he was being mocked by the establishment, considered a hopeless case.

"Play the game, Jason. They're trying to help you," became a frequent mantra I was growing sick of. I tried hard not to let my own concerns show, observing his fearful, sometimes tearful apprehension before and after meetings. Weighing up the fruits of the previous two meetings, I myself considered all of it futile. The meetings were generally repetitive and pointless, like *Groundhog Day*. Although this was a bittersweet chore, all other avenues had either been exhausted or extinguished entirely.

Arriving early, we sat in the car killing time, listening to the traffic from the High Street.

"Give it ten minutes, Jace," I said. "We'll still be early and it gives a good impression." I glanced at my watch then at my brother, who scowled at me like a brooding storm cloud through his cigarette smoke, less than convinced by the motivational tactics I'd been trying since we left.

He was lucky, I reminded him. George, the Trust worker

dealing with his case, seemed to have taken a liking to him. George discerned that Jason was a good egg and had vowed to do everything he could to try and help him achieve his goal. I wasn't entirely convinced what this 'everything' meant in practice, but for the time being I'd decided to go with the flow and see what opportunities unfolded.

"Remember that miserable old bat you used to see at the Job Centre, Jace?" I reminded him with a grin.

He shook his head and shuddered. They were truly the bad times. It was the way she asked Jason questions with her eyes fixed on a screen. She was talking to a case number, not the human being it represented. The robotic questioning was soul-destroying. 'What are you doing to find work? Have you applied for any jobs or done any work in the last two weeks? Blah blah blah.' These questions made me want to stand in front of her screen and ask her face-to-face if she had any job vacancies for a multi-addict who sees ghosts? With my brother shuffling in the seat in front of her, legs bobbing like a maniac, it was obvious that she perceived him as a hopeless bum happy to exist as a burden on the welfare system. Untrue and unfair.

The lack of understanding at the Job Centre was rivalled by their lack of support. The aftermath of those appointments there had left him downcast, as he thanked me for the lift and plodded mournfully across the road to his front door. I hated leaving him like that, when I knew he felt there was no point to any of it. I understood the mechanics of such despair. Inevitably they'd result in him seeking refuge with chemical support.

"You're better off with George. You know that," I reassured him now. Jason nodded his head and flicked his cigarette butt out of the window.

It was a testimony to George's good nature how he mustered the appetite to appear enthusiastic each time we met, which was always a tonic. Jason wasn't often at his best during appointments. It took a special quality to discern the good in a man as unravelled as my brother, and I believed George possessed it.

He was an even mannered, diligent type who, I felt, wanted to help all his clients. I sensed that between George and my brother was something more than occasional acquaintance, perhaps the flicker of fondness? He was the kind of well-meaning character you hoped to find in these places. However, there was a question mark hovering over him as regards how far he'd actually be able to help Jason.

Still, my scepticism about presenting Jason to an organisation I feared existed purely to manipulate unemployment figures was pacified for the time being. George shared my frustrations and appeared to have a plan on how to petition for better support. Proactive intervention I welcomed with open arms.

It was always hard to watch Jason's expression glaze over during discussions, staring at the wall or the floor as he recognised the problem case being discussed was himself. He was simply a voyeur to his own downfall. Sometimes this realisation felt insurmountable for him.

Since his short trial rehabilitation, he had lost contact with his original team and had been left alone to mend his ways. George understood the necessity to rekindle this relationship and get the support he needed if he was ever to get to the next stage of rehabilitation. George's motto became my own, as we agreed that Jason needed to be mentally able in order to work, particularly if he wanted to become a counsellor.

"There's no health without mental health," said George, smiling at Jason over his desk, his optimistic African face always displaying gentle empathy.

When George reviewed events since their last meeting, Jason's frustrations with the inertia of his other wellbeing appointments would boil over in angry outbursts.

"So how did last week's meeting go with your key worker, Jason?" George always asked the same question. Jason met his gaze.

"Same as always," he said blankly. "They say I have an hour then tell me they need to cut the time to half an hour."

Although his new key worker was a nice chap, the care team were woefully understaffed and appeared to be juggling multiple cases like chaotic circus clowns. His scheduled hour-long meetings, which he struggled to prepare himself for, were nearly always cut to fifteen or twenty minutes. The generic excuse offered every time was along the lines of 'unforeseen circumstances'. I felt as hopeless as him.

George shook his head and scribbled something in his notebook. There was a clue to George's own frustration in his tone as he stressed again that he had petitioned the mental health team to make sure Jason was back on their books and getting regular appointments.

"How the hell is he to remain motivated to rehabilitate if the care workers project such indifference?" I interjected. "I appreciate it may not be their intention but that's how it comes across."

Jason massaged the paint patch on his jeans, his eyes glazed and tearful. There was always the sense that everything within the welfare system was some half-hearted test. They gave a little, but waited to see what they got back before giving any more.

George and myself concurred. It wasn't realistic to expect Jason to be offered employment until his mind was in a better place. Jason pulled himself from his trance.

"The new care worker is quite a nice bloke, though," he suddenly piped up. "Only mid-thirties." Jason spontaneously looked more upbeat, as is his usual mood cycle. "Shame he doesn't have much time for me. He's already got me drinking proper cider, not that chemical stuff, and it's only half the alcohol."

Indeed, the new care worker knew his stuff. Having explained some simple methods to cut down Jason's intake, he'd managed to curb one of his longest reigning, most destructive habits. Jason had begun something of a renaissance where his health was concerned. As well as reducing his alcohol, he was cutting down on nicotine.

"Look, they've given me one of these." Jason rummaged through his trouser pockets excitedly before producing something and snapping it between his lips.

"What the hell is that? It looks like a tampon," I said. George also leaned across his table for a closer inspection.

"It's an NHS vape stick," Jason declared triumphantly from the side of his mouth. "They've given me some for free."

I'd seen more elaborate products in those early days of vaping and this was clearly their poorer relation, yet Jason was elated to have been deemed worthy of his freebie. Sucking hard, he produced a feeble cloud the size of a cotton-wool ball, which he blew towards me. George chuckled quietly before politely informing Jason he wasn't allowed to smoke in the office.

This made me realise how much my brother was willing to change his life and yet others didn't seem to recognise his new attitude. Surely he was now ripe for a full stint in rehab, a proper chance of change? If three months' half-hearted half-measures with a mentor affording half his allotted time had achieved this already, what could six months' rehabilitation harvest? Jason slid the vape stick back into his jacket pocket and looked downcast again.

"So you're still keen to become a counsellor, Jason?" asked George.

"Yeah. I think it's the only thing I could be good at."

But a few weeks later when we met George again, Jason was in an obstinate depression. George tried to ignore Jason's bobbing legs, which suddenly burst into life as he stared vacantly. It was a thankless task when he was like this. Some days he was gregarious and funny for an entire meeting, on others his moods swung like a metronome. Jason had become 'emotionally reticent' within ten minutes of being there. Having been optimistic about being able to help prevent others from squandering their lives, Jason appeared to have given up on optimism forever.

I believed that Jason could make a good counsellor if given the right nurturing. His warning message of where drugs could lead had undeniable credence, one that could definitely benefit other addicts. He was a nice guy, down on his luck and suffering some bad side effects as a result of his addictions. Everything about Jason added an authentic patina to his story, the haunted look of emaciated regret other troubled souls identified with. Even with his rough edges, when Jason felt upbeat he was fundamentally likeable to everyone who met him.

At the same time, dread spread over me as I considered my brother becoming a living testimonial of hopelessness and mental disrepair for others. It filled me with sadness to realise that Jason was so certain he'd never escape the clutches of addiction, he'd decided to parade them for all to see. A lump formed in my throat as I imagined him standing in front of a group of addicts in some young offenders' institution like an exhibit from a horror show. How long would he last doing that?

He'd always possessed a sensitive and caring nature, but if I pointed out the possible pitfalls of becoming a counsellor it would only upset the momentum of rehabilitation. The degree of comfort he'd gained when he'd first formed the brainwave that his life could serve some purpose for others was tangible. It had been good to see that rejuvenated zest for life in his blue eyes.

"I might meet a nice woman."

This was Jason's other aspiration, the ending of loneliness. My brother was a clumsy enigma when it came to women. In his darkest moments, women were pleasure objects. In his purest, he confided that by having a woman to love again he'd realise his greatest ambition. His early talent and promise as an artist had diminished with all his other faculties. Putting it in his own eloquent terms, whenever I endeavoured to lift his spirits, he'd look at me and say, "I'm really fucked now, aren't I?"

George slid a short questionnaire across the table.

"Could you fill this out, Jason?"

"What is it?" he asked glumly.

"Just some short questions to find out your general mood about things currently."

Each of the questions on the paper, George explained, required the participant to respond by grading their feelings on a scale of one to ten. Two short minutes' scribbling without lifting his head revealed my brother's lowly score as ones and twos for most questions. George considered his answers for a moment.

"You're not very optimistic today are you, Jason?" he asked sadly.

My brother shook his head in silence. I wanted to lean across and push his knees down to stop them jumping, or perhaps use some superglue on the soles of his boots. His legs had become increasingly frenetic as the meeting progressed. George rested his hands on the table and leaned forward.

"What would make you happier, Jason?" he asked. My brother shrugged his shoulders again.

"I think things will get better once the aliens arrive."

Jason looked at George with a deadpan expression. From George's dumbfounded face it was evident he'd not expected this answer. Should I intercede? I decided uncomfortably to go with the flow. Jason had to speak for himself whatever the outcome.

"Why would it be better when the aliens arrive, Jason?"

"They'd like me. They'd understand me better."

George and I exchanged bemused glances, recognising there was perhaps more than a little truth in my brother's statement. Jason's legs continued dancing without consent. George tapped his pen on the desk considering his next question. A thought occurred to me that if there were a questionnaire requiring me to grade George's patience, I'd definitely have given him ten. He studied Jason, searching for something to lift the mood.

"You really don't seem very happy all today." George was clearly struggling with where to go next.

"Well, I'm not very happy. I'm never really happy."

"What do you like to do to relax? Apart from drinking and drugs."

"I like taking coke."

Jason again fixed his eyes on George. He wasn't being contemptuous, but I could understand how one could interpret him as such. Jason liked George and knew he was trying. When he was waspish he was only being contemptuous of himself, with his inability to understand why he was like he was.

What was wrong with him anyway? The psychiatrists could never agree. A doctor our mother once worked for believed Jason showed a few classic symptoms of schizophrenia but had attributed these to psychosis through drug abuse, not an underlying condition. Other doctors he'd encountered within mental health care teams had debated this chicken and egg conundrum for years.

"What's the problem today, Jason? Something troubling you?" I asked the question that was teetering on George's tongue.

"I can't become a counsellor." Jason sniffed, turning his welling eyes to the floor.

He began incoherently explaining the full outcome of his last meeting with his care worker. He'd been full of gusto, saying how well he was doing with his alcohol intake as well as reducing his tobacco habit. It was open season for all his habits and he was culling them all one by one. Feeling the moment was ripe to announce his plans for the future, he'd shared with his care worker his desire to become a counsellor.

According to Jason, there was a pause as the man blinked in disbelief before shaking his head, cynically dismissing the notion without debate. The care worker would have known the full facts about how one became a counsellor, but his lack of empathy rocked me.

"I can't become a counsellor," Jason shook his head and slurred, "if I'm using anything. Even prescription drugs. Apparently, I haven't got a hope in Hell. I wouldn't even get a sniff at it."

The so-called care worker had taken an axe to Jason's hopes and aspirations. There must have been some other way of breaking the news other than to quash his hopes without compassion, offering up nothing to fill the chasm.

"That's… disappointing," I said feebly.

Jason nodded tearfully. It was strange the way he'd store important events inside like this and then suddenly regurgitate them. He's said nothing as he brooded in the car, as if he were readying himself to face this harsh truth with both of us.

"You need to set your sights on getting well first," said George. He clasped his hands on the table and gazed across the table compassionately. "Is there anything else you could set your sights on?"

"I have been thinking about that." Placing his palms on his knees, Jason wiggled in his chair. "You're probably going to laugh, though." He wore a serious frown and I felt the grip of apprehension.

"Come on, Jace. What do you think you could do?" I guiltily feared him answering that he wanted to work for me. Previous experience had proved that as unfeasible as a Chihuahua becoming a guard dog. Without a flicker of mischief or the faintest curl of a smile on his lips, he answered poker-faced.

"I want to be a ghostbuster." His face was convincing as he looked at us indignantly. "Well, I do see ghosts sometimes, don't I?"

I picked the phone up and dialled the number I'd been given by Jason with a feeling of sadness and exasperation.

"Hi, George. It's Marc King, Jason's brother."

"Hello, Marc. How are you?"

"To be honest, I'm a little confused," I said. George must have sensed the awkwardness, knowing there was a gripe coming his way. I could tell he was bracing himself. "I was talking to Jason today and he told me you're signing him back to the Job Centre?"

George cleared his throat to compose himself, his voice weak.

"The thing is, Jason has had his two years of support from the Trust. I've had to sign him back now."

"What good is that going to do? He needs help, not hate, George."

I realised I was out of line. But I feared that Jason's hopes of receiving nurturing to get him back to work were at an end.

"I've written a letter to explain Jason's condition for the Job Centre," George said in an effort to dilute my concerns. When I probed him further about who would be dealing with Jason's case and helping him back to work, his voice trailed off further. He stressed that it was important for Jason to keep his appointments with the Centre and with his key worker.

"I think it's more a case of them keeping their appointments with him, don't you think?" I mustered a sarcastic laugh.

"I'll phone from time to time to see how he's getting on," George tried to reassure me. I wondered how likely that would be. "Jason is always welcome to call me if he needs anything. That invitation extends to you also," he added politely.

It was hard to be magnanimous despite being thankful for the compassion George had extended to my brother during our time with him. My disappointment in him – and with the whole system – was obvious as I slammed my mobile down so hard I cracked the case.

We were back where we started. The harsh reality of life still rang true. If anyone was going to help Jason, it would have to be Jason himself.

18

THE RETURN

I sat in his dingy sitting room. I'd not seen him for a few weeks. Time had taken its toll on him, his unevenly shaved face had become increasingly gaunt, his eyes tired and red. There are times when I simply do not recognise Jason, when momentarily we become strangers.

"Anyway, Jace. We were talking about the cottage again, weren't we?" He looked at me seriously and nodded, almost apologetically, hands cupped on his lap.

"You know, when we started living there, I don't remember being frightened about seeing the old man again or the other things. Just startled." Jason looked pensive and thoughtful as he suddenly pondered his version of reality. "At first I was surprised when I saw it all, then it just became normal when I'd see things. You just accept stuff when you're a little kid, don't you? If nobody says anything you just accept they're supposed to be there."

"Not sure I could have done the same, Jason." I questioned how I could seriously consider the logic of his version of our story. We were talking about a ghost after all, an entity or something that I never saw but my brother clearly still believed in many years later. "I thought you were often scared inside the cottage, Jace?"

"I was, but not so much during those early days. It was just normal. As a little kid it I just thought it was a stranger who'd sometimes silently watch us." My brother snorted a laugh. "I probably thought it was some weird relative who'd not been introduced or something. I don't know. What intrigued me was why he was ignored by everyone."

When straight and contemplative like this, his stories gained plausibility.

"The fear came later when I was older and realised it wasn't normal." Hands still cupped on his lap, he stared at his boots searching for something. "I think that's why I played with my Action Men and toys so much. It kept my mind occupied."

I always remembered that facet about my brother, the avid way he'd entertain himself endlessly, often despite my every tactic to steal his attention for my own ends. Suddenly he stood, remembering something, his eyes wild. Spreading his arms wide, his long ragged coat opened like bat wings.

"I came in here the other night. You can ask my mate Martin if you want, he saw it. We were straight, honestly. I'd not had a thing for days, even a drink."

"Who's Martin? I regretted my question immediately, knowing Martin would be another hapless user and sadly not an entirely credible witness to whatever my brother was about to tell me.

"He's a good bloke. Anyway, it really made me jump when I opened the front door the other night. This black figure, darker than the darkness, darted across the room and disappeared upstairs." Jason swept his arms across the room like a magician. "Martin saw it and shouted that someone was in the house."

"Who was it?"

I looked around the gloomy room. Several sheets of newspaper stuck to the window acted as a makeshift curtain, rendering the small stairway entrance behind me a dark tunnel by mid-afternoon. Studying him, my sorrow was superseded by deeper curiosity. What was it Jason really experienced at times like this? The same old debate erupted, were these apparent visitors born from his early life as he claimed or from a syringe and a crack pipe? Harsh, but realistic logic.

"I know you think I'm mad, but I'm not, Marc." My brother shook his head at the floor miserably. "I told God to bring it back so I could see it properly and tell it to fuck off," he snorted vitriolically, his hands trembling with anger.

"God?"

"Yeah. I pray quite a lot these days."

This was a new revelation. My heart sank, it was worse than I thought. I could partly understand his reasoning for a belief in an entity that had tormented him, but a God that had left him like this?

"A few days later I was in bed asleep," he continued, "and suddenly something pulled my leg up into the air." Jason raised his hand in line with his hip. "I prayed for it to go and it went, just like that."

"That's quite a tale. I wond—"

"And I haven't told you about the frames the other day, have I?" he interrupted excitedly before sighing heavily and throwing the pillow from the armchair across the room to the sofa. Was he tired of everything? I felt a flood of empathy.

It was just getting light, he told me, when he'd come downstairs early that early autumn morning. Emerging from the stairs into the dark living room, he'd turned on the light and stood staring dumfounded at the once dreary paintwork. Now, there were over a hundred old-fashioned gilt frames all over the walls, all different sizes and hung perfectly straight with perfect gaps between them.

"Were you dreaming or tripping, Jace?"

"Neither," he snapped. "I'd had a few cans the previous night and gone to bed early as I didn't feel well."

"So what was in the frames?"

"I went to the kitchen and made a coffee hoping they'd be gone when I went back, but they were still there. All the frames were blank, just plain white paper inside." He shrugged. "I went upstairs and when I came down ten minutes later, they'd all gone."

This gave me another insight in my brother's mind,

often obliterated and blank, ready for the next instalment of inexplicable mayhem.

"Where are you at with your meds and the doctor?" I liked to check up on these to make sure he'd not been given anything new and problematic.

"I've got my most recent prescription here. The doc's really pleased with my progress. I hardly use most of this stuff now." Jason leaned back in his chair, stretching his sinewy legs fully out in front of him, and began frantically fishing with both hands inside his trouser pockets. "Here it is." Jason beamed. Holding the crumpled list in front of him he began reading his prescription with surprising pleasure as if reading a child a bedtime story.

"Buprenorphine 200 mg. One a day and the same..." He continued reading out the whole list to me, ending by insisting that he'd cut down on everything now, honestly. "The Pregabs too, even though I love 'em. They just keep you nice and calm all day."

So this was where mental health was at for most poor souls, a list of medicines to placate yourself with. I took the paper from him and studied it sadly.

"What about this one, the Haloperidol, four tablets a day? Have you cut down on those?" He looked me in the eye, his jocular sheen obliterated by something fearful.

"They're the ones I actually need," he snapped. Reaching over, he snatched the prescription back. "I can't reduce those. They help me stop seeing things."

Then suddenly, as always happens with my brother, he became someone else, an animated teenager talking about a documentary on dinosaurs in some Canadian lake that were seen in a time slip.

"So maybe there's a rational explanation for when I see things." He sat back, satisfied. I decided to give Jason's thought a curveball.

"You know I'm going to go down and visit the cottage again, Jace?"

"When?" he snapped, looking shocked, his forehead furrowed.

"Maybe this week or next, I'm not sure. I'm trying to psych myself up. I think I need to do it. Would you like to come, Jace?"

Taking a long sigh, Jason sat motionless in his favourite chair in a daydream and began to slowly shake his head.

"I'm curious but I'm not sure I'd want to go in." He paused. "Might make me feel worse."

Jason was sitting on his doorstep when I got back from revisiting the cottage. He was straight. He looked up at me full of uncertainty.

"What was it like?" he asked, like an impatient child. "Come in and have a cup of coffee, Marc. I want to hear about it."

It was mid-morning when I parked beside the gates to the gravelled driveway of Fir Tree Cottage. The forecast was for bright sunshine but a veil of mist inhibited my view of the lanes. Should I throw caution to the wind, just walk up the driveway and announce myself?

"Hi, I'm a complete stranger, just passing. I used to live here. Any chance I can come in?" Despite my apprehension I was bristling with excitement but reminded myself to calm down. The last thing I wanted was to unnerve the new occupants. There was, after all, something key I hoped to gain from my visit.

This was the place my brother believed to be the beginning of his torment. I tried imagining the figures he professed he'd seen when we first entered all those decades ago, one resembling an old man, another something vaguely female, the orbs he unexpectedly saw in various places.

Staring up the driveway, I remembered sitting in the lounge on cold winter evenings accompanied by an inexplicable sensation of unease. I never told my mother about it back then, knowing it would have only added to her mounting concerns. And there were things that even I, an agnostic, have never explained, like the voice that spoke to us in the garden once, that we thought must be God. We'd looked everywhere to find Him and I've never forgotten that voice.

That was what I hoped to gain from this visit, a healing of old memories and ultimately some answers about my brother.

It was incredible how time had stood still. Outside, the cottage appeared unchanged, lovingly maintained and friendlier than I remembered it yet still retaining its edgy quaintness. Everything normal. So why did I feel such a surge of uneasiness tying a knot in my stomach?

Perhaps I was resting too much hope on getting some final answers, some nugget of information that might help me understand the puzzle of my brother. I was looking for an end to this book about his life. And if I learned nothing, having found the courage to knock, I feared the emptiness it would leave. I'd have run out of avenues to help Jason.

I reflected on the happiness we'd experienced beyond the gates, the smells inside, the way the light danced through the windows. I suddenly wondered if the long rope swing was still there behind the rhododendrons. Then, what if I went inside and the place was unrecognisable? If the rambling cottage had become a million-pound modernised house, all my enduring memories from childhood would start fading.

We are, in so many ways, the sum of our own memories.

A loud knock on my window startled me and a surge of adrenalin shot through me. I looked up through the glass to see an old lady staring in at me, bemused and fierce.

"Are you lost?" she snapped.

I lowered the window and her repeated question came into the car as abruptly as her personality, firm and very middle class, her face parallel to mine. She wasn't crouching, she was just a tiny unrelenting package of incomparability.

"I'm not lost," I answered calmly. "I actually used to live here years ago."

"When?" she snapped, appraising me for signs of familiarity. "What's your surname?"

Christ, I thought, she's an ex-cop. I answered her obediently, trying to look innocent as I waited for her to retrieve a notebook from her back pocket. I was unprepared for the crack of her smile.

"You should go in and see them," she said. "They'd love it if you popped in and said hello." She turned and walked up the lane, disappearing into the mist like a ghost, without uttering another word. Obviously, I mean that metaphorically, I don't believe in ghosts. Ghosts are what people think they see when their minds play tricks on them. Sometimes, ghosts are what people see when they are unwell.

I stepped out of the car, closed the door and sucked in a lungful of clean air before heading towards the gate. My stomach did cartwheels again as the knot tied an extra coil. At the gate, I pulled up the latch and a dog appeared from nowhere. It was one of those big old English sheepdogs, clipped and groomed so its large doleful eyes peered up from under its neatly chiselled fringe like the eyelid windows of the cottage. An inspirational choice of breed, I thought.

Now, I love dogs but this wasn't my front garden anymore. Nevertheless she appeared relaxed so I opened the gate and she stared at me with optimistic curiosity before bolting through a gap in a hedge leading onto the front lawn. The hedge was a new addition, perfectly placed to block the view of the entire cottage from the lane. I'd only walked three or four steps before the dog reappeared with a toy hanging from her jaw, a ball on a rope, her rear end wagging enthusiastically. It appeared that my new four-legged friend was not only welcoming me back but also wanted to play.

It was becoming like old times.

I continued up the drive without a clue what words would follow after I'd uttered my initial nervous greeting. I noticed that both the garage lean-to and my father's work cabin had been removed and I felt a twinge of sadness. Both outbuildings had provided imperative crawl space and made the path behind them feel secret and undiscovered by adults, our route to escape unhappiness whenever it hunted us. I carried on up the short steps to the patio. As I glanced back across the garden, I realised that somehow a part of me had never left the place.

The dog stayed close, circling my legs and still waving its rear end expectantly as I walked to the porch door and knocked two times. It was only a few seconds before the door opened, a few seconds that felt like minutes, as every structured sentence I'd tried rehearsing left my mind completely. The women who answered looked out with surprise, first at me and then at the dog.

"Well, Cassie seems to have found a friend," she said, smiling and dumfounded.

"Hello. Sorry to bother you. I hope you don't mind me intruding…" Words tumbled out like a waterfall and the women watched me quite baffled. Finally, I managed, "Um, I used to live here when I was a child and I was parked outside when one of your neighbours suggested I should come in…" The perfect alibi. Blame it on the old lady.

"Oh. Who was that, I wonder?" The women placed her index finger to her lip thoughtfully. I described the tiny woman in the lane but the women shook her head blankly. "We don't have much to do with the people around here. It's the area we've come for." I nodded my understanding, it was precisely our experience of the cottage while we lived there. "It's a bit snooty round here to be honest," she continued, running her gaze along the perimeter of the fence behind at the surrounding lanes.

Her husband joined us at the door, moving close to his wife in the darkness of the porch. I realised with a start that weirdly he bore an uncanny resemblance to my late grandfather. I introduced myself.

"Yes, I remember your surname on the deeds." She smiled and a wave of relief washed over me. We'd become connected. "Would you like to come in?"

I focused my curiosity on the inside of the cottage, looking around the lounge as if I were casing the joint. It looked recently decorated and although brighter it was mostly how I remembered it from all those years ago, the same colours and smells. The cottage still preserved its essence of the past although the fireplace looked smaller, more modern.

Secretly I longed to be granted free rein to inspect the whole place. The twin wooden doors opening to the stairs were still present and I lingered, looking at the doors like a hopeful pup. The owners watched me quietly as I studied the place self-consciously, fearing I might have already outstayed my welcome. I pointed to the open door that led down to what used to be the garage.

"That was our playroom." The couple smiled silently as I continued looking around with wonderment, memories flooding back. They observed me like patient parents letting a five year-old loose in their house. "Can I take a look?" I asked.

"Of course," the woman said.

As they followed me down the short steps, I was caught in a moment of childlike excitement. Although there was different furniture, each individual room of the cottage had somehow retained its distinct scent. The playroom was always colder than the rest of the cottage, coupled with a faint whiff of mossy dampness filtering from the garden.

I gazed outside as a vivid reconstruction played out in my head of my brother and I scurrying across the lawn in the summer, readying ourselves to embark on another mission. I thought about our games where we always played the same fictitious characters, crouching behind the low brick wall flanking the driveway, stashes of gravel and stones stored ready to pelt imaginary assailants. During the colder months we'd huddle behind the wall to shield ourselves from the wind that billowed across the open garden, stubbornly refusing to seek refuge inside.

One particular day, some years after we'd moved in, I remembered well. Jason and I sat on the wall of the patio, looking across the garden dismally at the short lifeless stump protruding from the earth, all that was left of the towering fir tree. Men had come one morning to remove it from our lives despite our protests. Jason had consoled me as tears trickled down my face.

He told me it would all be alright and we'd find 'another best tree' to climb.

"Do you remember anything strange happening when you lived here?"

The woman's words broke into my memories like a knife. I faced her, not quite believing what she'd just asked. The couple observed me with a look of intense expectation and everything I'd locked away in a compartment of my mind marked 'Things not to ask the new owners of Fir Tree Cottage' spilled out.

I felt excited. Maybe there was an explanation for my brother to be had from this place after all.

"Well, the place was exorcised before we moved in," I said with a disbelieving smile. There was no reaction, just poker-faced expressions. Was I telling them something they already knew? Had I blown it and they were now thinking they'd let a crazy man in their house? Yet the man appeared unfazed, his head angled as if evaluating my response. "I guess you may already know about the history of this cottage?" I asked hopefully.

"We've had friends stay in this room," the woman replied. "They found themselves desperate to leave in the middle of the night."

My visit was becoming more than I'd bargained for. My jaw hung loose in disbelief. Noticing the sofa bed, I idly wondered how much I could pay them to let me stay here for a night.

"What I can say is that when I lived here I never actually saw anything, but I remember many times feeling unsettled. There were times when I'd run downstairs from my room feeling I was being watched, despite the room being empty," I disclosed. The woman nodded knowingly. "I have to admit I was curious whether you'd experienced anything like that since moving here."

The women smiled at her husband and explained that they'd always felt happy in the cottage. Accepted. Their son, however, couldn't wait to flee the nest and had felt uneasy within the walls. It was time for me to fess up, I told myself. I followed them back up the stairs and into the lounge where the couple sat on the sofa and I took a chair by the window. The man remained quietly contemplative.

"Actually, I've started writing a book about my brother. A lot of it revolves around the experiences he had here." They looked back at me pensively. Had I said too much? "He's had continued drug and alcohol dependency most of his life, starting when he was fourteen. He also maintains that the apparitions that plague him originated here."

I felt certain I'd given away too much information and they'd think I'd visited like a snooping hack looking for gems with which to finish my story. Paranoia crept over me like cold mist. I felt vulnerable for surrendering this information, stuff I'd rarely talked about and had certainly not intended to during this visit. Nevertheless, the couple appeared unfazed, particularly the woman's husband.

"Regardless of whether he's straight, which is a rarity..." I carried on with a feeble laugh, "...or going through a period of complete oblivion, his story remains the same. He believes something followed him from here."

"It sounds," the husband spoke for the first time, his brow furrowed thoughtfully, "as though he's suffered some kind of psychosis. Possibly drug-induced."

I'd always wanted to agree with this logic but Jason's difficulties had started at a very early age, before he'd experimented with drugs. Although he was always a sensitive person, I knew he'd become gradually stranger since we moved here. As I understood it, he'd taken drugs to escape his torments. I looked the man in the eye.

"You sound like a psychiatrist," I said flippantly.

"I am a psychiatrist," he stated calmly and efficiently, looking at me with a gentle, no-nonsense expression.

It's unnerving to realise you've obliviously unearthed your life story to a shrink, like waking from a dream to discover you've not only been sleepwalking but you're also naked.

"That's a bit of a coincidence," I said, desperately trying to make friendly small talk. "My company is actually refurbing part of a psychiatric hospital next week."

"Which hospital?" he asked with considered curiosity. I told him the name of the place and he looked at me thoughtfully again as the room filled with a tangible silence. "I used to be the chief psychiatrist there," he said.

There was no denying this peculiar coincidence and it hit me like an epiphany. If this man was a senior authority on mental health, he'd know a lot of psychiatrists. I'd inadvertently discovered a possible ally to point me in the right direction with my brother's care. And now I was preoccupied by the possibility he could provide helpful information. Maybe he had a better understanding than all the other shrinks Jason had encountered in his life.

Here was the first warm, bona fide mental health expert I'd interacted with, and he was living in our old cottage. We were practically related. This was the real reason I was supposed to visit: destiny had a plan.

"The chief psychiatrist at Jason's hospital finally gave him a statement after years of us trying to get one," I told them. "He stated that his paranoid schizophrenia was possibly attributed to substance abuse."

The man listened intently as I explained, however, that this statement had been issued without medical consensus on Jason. It seemed to me that, with all the cutbacks, the infirm and vulnerable were bundled into the same equation as the feckless. They'd all become government targets needing to be persecuted into work, not understood. There was no resource for understanding. The statement had simply effectively removed Jason from the growing list of those deemed work-dodging parasites, but left him without support.

"Has your mother ever wanted to come back and look around again?" the woman asked quickly, perhaps fearing the conversation would descend into a political debate. "You're welcome to bring her down."

"She'd love to visit. Although she admits the cottage holds lots of unhappy memories. But I'm sure she'd love to look around the old place. That's very kind of you."

I was telling a big white lie. Mum would never want to set foot in the cottage again unless I could coerce her. She considered the place as the alpha and omega of her own unhappiness, and the likelihood of her returning was remote. She blamed herself for everything that went wrong during our childhood as if it was her decision alone to drag us to the countryside. She'd forgotten too readily the positive benefits for us of living here as children, the freedom and scenic beauty that instilled our love of the countryside.

Still, the woman had handed me the golden ticket to a second visit, if I could convince Mum to come with me.

"It would be interesting to talk to her and see what she remembers." The women now stood, looking about the room as if imagining my mother entering again after over forty years' absence. A part of me felt frustrated, she clearly wanted to talk to the mother, not the child. What specifically was it she wanted to know?

By their body language of polite smiles and stalling conversation I understood that my visit was at an end, the meter had expired.

"Thank you so much for letting me take a look around. It's very kind of you." The husband shook my hand and I looked at his familiar face, feeling that we still had unfinished business to discuss.

I felt a pang of regret as the woman opened the door. I was leaving them with a tarnished depiction of my brother. I'd not done the man behind the madness any justice. I'd not told them how Jason was honest and overly appreciative of the smallest kindnesses. How if someone asked him for a place to stay and food to eat, he'd offer whatever he had readily, which now was practically nothing. I toyed with the notion of quickly telling them how my brother would give you his last penny if he thought he was helping you. Or how much Jason appreciated it when I didn't insist on a receipt from the cash machine. Simple acts of trust made my brother beam with happiness. He was a person with morals and credibility.

But the time for stories had passed. I walked along the patio feeling slightly ashamed. The fresh air sobered me as I grappled how best to initiate another conversation about Jason next time I visited. On the driveway I glanced behind, the couple watching me from the front door as I walked through the gate. I consoled myself that hopefully another opportunity would arise for me to explain my brother better.

Beside my car, I turned to face the garden savouring its scent and remembering the child. My now grown-up brother had changed from the sensitive, quirky kid to a man who now lived his life in relative squalor. Afraid he would be thrown out by the landlord if he made a fuss about his heating not working. He'd rather sit huddled under a blanket enduring the cold winter months than complain. Jason felt unworthy and was scared of being perceived as a problem tenant, a parasite.

I couldn't bring myself to leave quite yet. Looking towards the cottage rekindled an obscure memory of Jason's squinting gaze fixed high above him on a branch where a robin sang. The garden had been full of wonder for him then. How had it happened that those days of joy were now replaced by fear of apparitions springing from nowhere?

Looking up into the gently swaying boughs I relished the birdsong again. The fresh countryside fragrance always sends me back to our childhood. Despite the sadness and upheaval we experienced in those younger years, I felt at home here. At the slope by the rhododendrons it seemed as though at any moment our childhood would replay like a movie. Jason and I would be doing tandem jumps from the rope swing, daring to leave it longer and longer before releasing ourselves onto the gathered beds of crispy autumn leaves.

Would Jason come back here? He was definitely curious

although also uneasy about the cottage. How would it make him feel, revisiting the garden after all these years with memories ready to ambush him from behind every shrub or maze of ferns? What would it be like for him to go back inside? Would it prove to be a terrible idea or help him? I felt an urgency to make it happen soon before time ran out, as it has a habit of doing for everyone.

The sun feathered my face and the warmth of the day began making an appearance. Above, the birds grew louder, hopping across branches and darting like arrows. Cassie lay contentedly perusing the garden in the middle of the lawn, eyes half-closed and at ease with my presence.

Sometimes my own spontaneity takes me by surprise. I turned and lifted the latch on the gate and stepped back onto the driveway, hoping the shrubs on the bottom lawn would obscure me sufficiently. Alone in the garden again, I felt as mischievous as a child. A lump rose in my throat as another recollection appeared from the past, so lucid it almost became a vision.

On the lawn I saw my brother squinting through soft sunlight into the face of a holy man in flowing black robes, a kind man who understood hope and humility. He smiled into Jason's face, ruffling the top of his head playfully. My brother surveyed him, our football in the crook of his skinny arm, wearing that awkward uncertain smile of his. In the stillness of my memory, I was a voyeur to an unspoken understanding between them.

I was reminded of a brother who made an appearance every once in a while without warning, and always when you'd lost all hope of ever seeing him again.

EPILOGUE

Perhaps the biggest epidemic the world faces today is mental illness. Consideration, understanding and connection are the first pivotal points for any intercession. These are the cheapest resources we can all share in abundance, to prevent another person's lifetime of turmoil.

The lack of professional resources is an ongoing struggle. Yet the more awareness there is about mental health issues, the more resources will have to increase or the epidemic will spiral out of control.

A friend of mine who does outreach community work through a local church knows most of the troubled souls in a south London borough. Some he's met through the food banks, others through face-to-face counselling. He listens and offers understanding and in many cases this interaction has led people to live more fulfilled lives, even enabling some to get professional help.

As we walked our dogs around the park one morning, we discussed the value of human understanding and connection and he shared a story about a kid that once lived in his street.

Sam was a polite boy. Everyone in the street liked him. He was courteous, helpful, keen to engage in conversation, in many ways a perfect eleven year-old lad. Sam was a shining example of youth until he went to secondary school and the doors shut behind him. Once inside the school walls he felt imprisoned and anxious like a wild animal. He became the most disruptive kid in the school, in fact the most disruptive kid in all the schools he subsequently went to and was excluded from. He threatened violence to teachers and other rowdy pupils. He was labelled a no-hoper, destined for prison or worse.

My friend had engaged with him not long after his family moved in. He said that when Sam's mother had confided all of this, the revelations had shocked him.

Everything changed when a diligent occupational therapist sat Sam in a quiet room and listened, most importantly understood. The old guard of teachers had labelled him with 'naughty child syndrome' when in fact Sam had severe ADHD. This is a very real condition. Sam was a lucky one, someone noticed and took action. He just needed that understanding, a small classroom, and the rest he took care of himself. He soared.

"You should see him now, Marc," my friend said. "Eleven years later and he's one of the top paramedics in the country. He's flying, he's got a house, a partner. It's an incredible transformation."

I told Jason this story and, true to form, at first he got very excited and then almost immediately quite sad.

"I could have been a great drugs counsellor, Marc. I'm really good at talking to people about those sorts of things." My brother looked full of regret, thinking about the care workers that had put an end to his dream. "Maybe, if people read your book about my life, it might help others?" Jason smiled, his eyes full of hope, regret and empathy.

If you have enjoyed this book...

Local Legend is committed to publishing the very best spiritual writing, both fiction and non-fiction. You may also enjoy:

THE SOUL CAVE
Sandra Francis (ISBN 978-1-910027-57-8)

Every one of us, Sandra believes, has far greater ability and energy than we realise and in everyday life we only use a small part of our extraordinary minds. We each have the power to create the happy, fulfilled and peaceful lives our souls crave and deserve. Yes, life has many challenges, but we can rise above them and turn them to our advantage, healing the pain of past events and forming new, better relationships. And it's never too late...

Sandra is proof of this. Despite illness and trauma, in middle age she set out on a spiritual path of loving acceptance, forgiveness and gratitude that completely changed her life. In this beautifully written book, she shows us all the way.

PAST LIFE HEALING
Judy Sharp (ISBN 978-1-910027-52-3)

Do we live many lives – and could trauma of the past still be affecting our health and wellbeing here and now? The author was completely healed of her own severe claustrophobia in one session and now has decades of professional experience helping others with issues from fear of flying to stubborn weight gain. This truly eye-opening book gives many evidential case studies, alongside a wealth of information about the concept of past lives across history and different cultures, as well as details of the extensive research carried out in this field.

Winner of the national *Spiritual Writing Competition.*
"A fascinating insight… highly recommended!"
Wishing Shelf Book Awards

LOVE, DEATH AND BEYOND
Helen Ellwood (ISBN 978-1-910027-51-6)

Helen had always been almost afraid of living, believing that mere dark oblivion awaited her in the end. Trained in medical sciences and having rejected religious beliefs, she often felt terrified. But Beryl the hamster changed everything when her soul rose from her body at death, and Helen was shocked into opening herself to the spiritual and the numinous. The paranormal experiences came one after another then and it was soon clear that the human mind was far more powerful, and consciousness far more enduring, than she had imagined. Every reader will identify with the author's doubts and fears, and be inspired by this beautifully written memoir.

Winner of the national *Spiritual Writing Competition.*
and Bronze Medal in *The Wishing Shelf Book Awards*
"…compelling… intriguing…" with score 94%

GHOSTS OF THE NHS
Glynis Amy Allen (ISBN 978-1-910027-34-9)

It is rare to find an account of interaction with the spirit world that is so wonderfully down-to-earth! The author simply gives us one extraordinary true story after another, as entertaining as they are evidential. Glynis, an hereditary medium, worked for thirty years as a senior hospital nurse in the National Health Service, mostly in A&E wards. Almost on a daily basis, she would see patients' souls leave their bodies escorted by spirit relatives or find herself working alongside spirit doctors – not to mention the Grey Lady, a frequent ethereal visitor! A unique contribution to our understanding of life, this book was an immediate bestseller.

Winner of the SILVER MEDAL in the national
Wishing Shelf Awards.
"What a fascinating read. The author has a way of putting across a story that is compelling and honest… highly recommended!"

SPIRIT REVELATIONS
Nigel Peace (ISBN 978-1-907203-14-5)

With descriptions of more than a hundred proven prophetic dreams and many more everyday synchronicities, the author shows us that, without doubt, we can know the future and that everyone can receive genuine spiritual guidance for our lives' challenges. World-renowned biologist Dr Rupert Sheldrake has endorsed this book as "…vivid and fascinating… pioneering research…"

A national runner-up in *The People's Book Prize* awards.

HAUNTED BY PAST LIVES
Sarah Truman (ISBN 978-1-910027-13-4)

When Sarah's partner told her that she had murdered him, she took little notice. After all, dreams don't mean anything, do they? But Tom's recurring and vividly detailed dreams demanded to be investigated and so the pair embarked upon thorough and professional historical research, uncovering previously unknown facts that seemed to lead to only one simple conclusion: past lives are true! Yet even that was not the end of their story, for they had unwittingly lifted the lid on some dramatic supernatural phenomena...

THE HOUSE OF BEING
Peter Walker (ISBN 978-1-910027-26-4)

Acutely observed spiritual verse by a master of his craft, showing us the mind, the body and the soul of what it is to be human in this glorious natural world. A linguist and a priest, the author takes us deep beneath the surface of life and writes with sensitivity, compassion and, often, with searing wit and self-deprecation. This is a collection the reader will return to again and again.

A winner of the national *Spiritual Writing Competition*.

TAP ONCE FOR YES
Jacquie Parton (ISBN 978-1-907203-62-6)

This extraordinary book offers powerful evidence of human survival after death. When Jacquie's son Andrew suddenly committed suicide, she was devastated. But she was determined to find out whether his spirit lived on, and began to receive incredible yet undeniable messages from him on her mobile phone... Several others also then described deliberate attempts at spirit contact. This is a story of astonishing love and courage, as Jacquie fought her own grief and others' doubts in order to prove to the world that her son still lives.

"A compelling read." The national *Wishing Shelf Book Awards*.

ODD DAYS OF HEAVEN
Sandra Bray (ISBN 978-1-910027-17-2)

If you feel that you've lost the joy in your life and are not sure where you're going, this book is written for you. Sandra knows those feelings all too well. Rocked by mid-life events, she refused to be a victim of circumstances and instead resolved to treat them as opportunities for change and growth. She looked for a spiritual 'guide book' to offer her new thoughts and activities for each day, but couldn't find one – so she wrote it! In this book, and her sequel *Even More Days of Heaven*, we find almost four hundred brilliantly researched suggestions, sure to life our spirits.

Runner-up in the national *Spiritual Writing Competition*.

Local Legend titles are available worldwide
as paperbacks and eBooks.
Further details and extracts of these and many
other beautiful books for the Mind, Body and Spirit
may be seen at

https://local-legend.co.uk

www.ingramcontent.com/pod-product-compliance
Lightning Source LLC
LaVergne TN
LVHW051548080426
835510LV00020B/2902